ethics in medicine

ethics in medicine

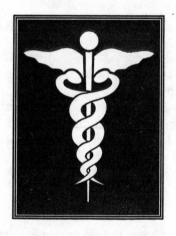

Milton D. Heifetz, M.D.

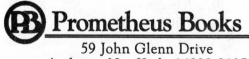
Prometheus Books
59 John Glenn Drive
Amherst, New York 14228-2197

Published 1996 by Prometheus Books

00 99 98 97 96   5 4 3 2 1

Library of Congress Cataloging-in-Publication Data

Heifetz, Milton D., 1921–
    [Easier said than done]
    Ethics in medicine / Milton D. Heifetz.
        p.   cm.
    Originally published under title: Easier said than done,
Prometheus Books, 1992.
    Includes bibliographical references and index.
    ISBN 1–57392–073–8 (paper)
    1. Medical ethics. I. Title.
R724.H42   1996
174'.2—dc20   96–17892
                                                            CIP

Printed in the United States of America on acid-free paper

To Betsy

Contents

Introduction 9

Acknowledgments 15

1. A Concept of Ethics 17

2. General Problems in Application 39

3. The Doctor-Patient Relationship 45

4. The Right of Self-Determination 71

5. Suicide 107

6. Abortion 123

7. The Tragic Newborn 143

8. Euthanasia 159

9. Human Experimentation 173

8   Contents

10. The Ethics of Medical Triage:
    Allocation and Rationing of Health Care   197

Summary   213

Appendices

    A. Discussion of Mastery   215

    B. Discussion of Privacy   219

    C. Example of Durable Power of Attorney   225

    D. Recommendations Regarding Fetal Research   227

    E. The Belmont Report of the
       National Commission for the Protection
       of Human Subjects of Biomedical and
       Behavioral Research   233

    F. The Foundation of Human Rights   251

Index   253

Introduction

Ethics speaks primarily to the right and wrong in human relationships. It is from the study of ethics and, consequently, a better understanding of moral principles, that society may hope to enhance the sense of tolerance, fairness, compassion, and sensitivity to another's pain and thereby improve aspects of human behavior that place humans in a separate niche in biological history.

Ethical questions, especially as they apply to medicine, have become common topics of discussion during the past twenty years. Bitter disputes have arisen regarding abortion, suicide, human experimentation, as well as the management of the dying patient and the severely disabled newborn. These issues do not lead to gentle, dispassionate discourse. They are loaded with such emotion that it is sometimes difficult to look at them in a detached manner. This is especially true in a society that aims to be secular, but which is strongly influenced by religious doctrines. Because of the confusion surrounding these disputes, the medical profession has developed ethics and human experimentation committees to help resolve these complex issues, which are part of the daily life of physicians and other health-care workers. Within the past twenty years these committees have become standard

9

fixtures in every major hospital in America. Nationwide seminars on patient rights and ethics have become commonplace, and medical students are, for the first time, being exposed to classes in ethics alongside their classes in medicine and surgery.

The complexity of ethical dilemmas and resultant clamor will become more bewildering as technology continues to advance. We are facing a time when an egg and a sperm with desirable genetic attributes will be brought together in a Petri dish, nourished until transplanted into the uterus of a future mother, all according to parameters spelled out in a computer containing lists of potential donors. The ethical issues surrounding a surrogate mother are simple compared to those that all of us will face in the future. It has become a moot point whether ethically we should or should not move along certain potentially dangerous lines of research. The fact is that we will continue all areas of research and thus will be in need of greater understanding of ethics involved in the application of our knowledge. In order to clarify the fundamental premises upon which ethical decisions must rest, we need to stand back and assess our situation, free from the burdens of tradition, dogma, or gut reaction that limit our thinking.

As this volume progresses we will see the development of four principles that I believe are fundamental to making moral judgments. These principles are not peculiar to medical ethics. As K. D. Clouser so pointedly expresses it, "Medical ethics is no big deal . . . it is simply ethics applied to a particular area of our lives . . . it is the 'old ethics' trying to find its way around in new, very puzzling circumstances."[1]

I have made decisions as a neurosurgeon for forty years in often tragic and anguishing situations. I have sat on human experimentation and hospital ethics committees for many years. During innumerable discussions within these committees, it has become apparent that a strong grasp of fundamental principles is all too often clouded by irrelevancies that tend to confuse the decision-making process. The dilemma of separating gut reaction from dispassionate decision making is a constant for all physicians. A better understanding of how to navigate the ethical road when there are conflicts of interest for both the patient and the doctor may make these dilemmas, which are compounded by the physician's fear of lawsuits from survivors as well as patients, less disturbing. Defensive medicine with its excess ordering of tests has become an unpleasant way of life for most physicians. Dishonesty, whether perpetrated by patients or physicians, is commonplace. A patient asks for an extension of disability that is not medically warranted. Does the physician say no, thereby possibly antagonizing and losing the patient, or does the insurance company or taxpayer pay the unnecessary bill? How can we avoid this?

This work is an attempt to more clearly delineate the pertinent factors necessary for decision making in various troublesome areas in medicine. My primary intent is to help those who must make decisions involving difficult medical ethical problems, especially physicians, nurses, hospital ethics committees, and medical students. It should also prove relevant to policy makers who struggle to legislate sound rules of conduct in medical decisions.

Most of these problems have been discussed by many before me. The richness of this literature is immense. In the following chapters I will describe some of the dilemmas surrounding moral issues in medicine and how the physician and patient together can work toward solving them. In the process I hope that I will have achieved a crystallization of basic principles that will serve as a solid foundation for evaluating ethical dilemmas.

The eight topics I plan to discuss do not cover all areas of medical ethics; for instance, genetic engineering and psychosurgery are not addressed. The topics have been selected for three specific reasons: they are of great public interest; they are areas in which I, as well as most physicians, have been intimately involved or concerned; and, in addition, they serve as excellent vehicles to demonstrate the principles underlying medical ethics.

It is not my intention to, nor can any physician, deal with all the nuances that may arise when those who practice medicine are faced with the ambiguous aspects of medical ethical issues. I seek instead to establish the basic framework upon which ethical decisions should be based. The chapters are therefore not designed to be in-depth discussions of each topic since many books have already been written about each of them. Rather, my hope is to demonstrate how the basic ethical framework may be applied within the confines of uncertainty. It is only after a thorough understanding of fundamental principles, their interrelationships and their hierarchy, that subtle gray areas can become less troublesome. Physicians can then approach ethical problems with more security and, since they are tinged with elements of anguish, less emotional confusion.

The approach I have used is to try to establish general principles that may then be applied to different situations rather than the commonly used case study method in which the principles are thought to emerge from a case-by-case analysis. In chapter 1, I have derived, from an attitude common to all people and from religious and secular philosophy, a set of fundamental principles that can be used to clarify ethical questions and are consonant with human nature. By using this framework and extrapolating from it when necessary, we should be able to evaluate virtually any medical ethical situation. Safety, respect for the patient, and consistency in application will be the paramount elements guiding this discussion.

Subsequent chapters will attempt to apply the ethical principles developed in chapter 1 to specific controversial areas of medicine.

NOTE

1. K. Danner Clouser, "Medical Ethics: Some Uses, Abuses, and Limitations," *The New England Journal of Medicine* 293, no. 8 (August 21, 1975): 384.

Acknowledgments

I have been very fortunate in the quality of help I received during the development of this manuscript. I had the privilege, while a visiting scholar at Oxford University during the 1991 Trinity term, to have the first chapter "A Concept of Ethics," which is the foundation upon which the book rests, critiqued by John C. B. Glover, John Gray, Ralph C. S. Walker, and Bernard A. O. Williams. Their dedication and meticulous reading of this chapter resulted in constructive criticisms of immense value in clarifying my thoughts. I also wish to acknowledge my debt of gratitude to a number of scholars who have reviewed various drafts of the complete manuscript and have been most helpful in their criticism and suggestions: George Annas, Charles H. Baron, Peter Mcl. Black, Sissela Bok, James Childress, Arthur Dyck, Jay Katz, Irwin C. Lieb, Mark Moore, Derek Parfit, Lynn Petersen, Mike Rie, and Dennis Thompson. I would also like to express my thanks to my editor Steven Mitchell, who has been so perceptive and helpful. Last but not least, I am grateful to my wife, my children, and my brother and sister, who read and reread multiple versions of this manuscript.

Whatever flaws or conclusions there may be are entirely my own responsibility.

This work has been supported by a grant from the Deutsch Foundation of Los Angeles.

1

A Concept of Ethics

The words "ethics" and "morals," through common usage (and in the present context), are often used interchangeably. We speak of an ethical person as being a moral person. Moral issues arise whenever human action or inaction affects others. Customs and values reflect the moral underpinning of a society. Laws that mandate behavior patterns should, but do not always, reflect ideal moral values. Morality speaks to what is right or wrong in human relationships,[1] how we should treat others and how others ought to treat us, how each individual should behave in a social order, and how that social order should relate to each of us.

The understanding of right and wrong and the acceptable means of achieving goals, as reflected in the behavior of the adult individual, are based upon values inculcated during childhood according to the general and specific values of parents and society. As William Frankena expresses it, "Morality starts as a set of culturally defined goals and of rules governing achievement of the goals, that are more or less external to the individual and imposed on him."[2]

Since there are significantly different ethical values

and therefore different codes of behavior among the diverse cultures in the world, the question arises whether a framework exists from which realistic moral principles may be derived that diverse groups may use when they relate to one another, regardless of the value differences among them. I believe such a framework does exist. The task is to identify it. But how do we begin?

An ethical format may be derived from several approaches. The primary frame of reference might be religious dogma, reason based upon assumptions, or fundamental universal attributes of humans that are independent of cultural patterns or beliefs.

Ideally moral principles regardless of their derivation should be:

1. prescriptive in the sense of giving direction as to how we should act;
2. proscriptive in the sense of suggesting what would be unacceptable behavior;
3. potentially applicable to all areas of the human condition;
4. acceptable to diverse cultures and thereby have universal application;
5. suggestive that adherence to them generally functions to the long-term benefit of the individual and society;
6. in harmony with human nature.

THREE POTENTIAL FRAMEWORKS

Religion as a Frame of Reference

Religious faith has been and still is a major factor in influencing ethical values. I would like to delineate two aspects of religious thought pertinent to this discussion:

(1) religious dogma and (2) religious philosophy. Religious dogma is a formally stated and authoritatively proclaimed doctrine of a given church. Although dogma is open for discussion, the validity of the dogma is not subject to challenge. One is expected to accept as a matter of belief the validity of that dogma. Religious philosophy, on the other hand, investigates general principles of human nature, conduct, and religious belief from the point of view of the church.

If religious dogma were to be accepted as the foundation of ethics, many questions would inevitably arise, such as: which doctrine is to be followed and which interpretation of that doctrine is to be respected? In a pluralistic society, with many faiths and points of view, severe controversies would arise. The rights and wrongs of abortion and suicide are obvious cases in point.

Although religious freedom may be a paramount value in our society, the memory of the Dark Ages, Galileo, Spinoza, and the Inquisition alerts us to the dangers of religious dogma and especially to fanatical interpreters of that dogma. In the unswerving belief in the truth of dogma lies the seed of fanaticism and intolerance. A free, secular, pluralistic society is probably less prone to erosion of freedoms if there is a strong separation of church and state. With due respect to formal religious groups, it is much safer for the preservation of freedom if the responsibility for the formation and maintenance of a code of ethics is secular in character.

However, religious philosophy contains great wisdom that is edifying to all people. There is little in the way of basic moral precepts that has not already been expressed in one form or another in the literature of the great religions.

Reason as a Frame of Reference[3]

The second possible frame of reference is that of reason. The path that reasoning will take and the subsequent conclusions drawn follow directly from the initial assumptions, as well as the quality of the subsequent reasoning. Even a reasonable approach may lead to arbitrary and somewhat idiosyncratic conclusions. An extreme example would be to start with the primary assumption that the purpose of life is to be happy and then to conclude that any action enhancing one's happiness is acceptable, regardless of its effect upon others. A frame of reference for morality must rest upon a more solid foundation.

Universal Attribute as a Frame of Reference

My approach is to utilize a universal human attribute, which stems from our biological inheritance—the desire to avoid harm—as the framework upon which I hope to base moral principles that are applicable to many cultures. This effort is made with full awareness that Kant believed such a task would be impossible because it could not lead to what *ought* to be done morally.[4] We will see if this impression is valid. But first I must acknowledge the cautious words of Peter Singer:

> The suggestion that an aspect of human ethics is universal, or nearly so, in no way justifies that aspect of human ethics. Nor does the suggestion that a particular aspect of human ethics has a biological basis do anything to justify it.[5]

I appreciate this sentiment since the human animal has to a great extent moved away from many natural-selection forces. Second, I recognize that just because something exists in subhuman mammals does not make it necessarily applicable to human society. Because some female monkeys may adopt an orphan monkey does not mean that what looks like altruism can be used to validate altruism in people, any more than the brutal killing of a baby gorilla by the new mate of a widowed gorilla could recommend the same behavior for humans. It is apparent that what is natural is not necessarily good. Cancer is an obvious example. It is also obvious that people may control their inherited mammalian impulses. Individuals readily risk their lives to climb mountains, or sacrifice themselves for an abstract cause in spite of the intense inherited impulse to preserve life.

Although Singer's comment is certainly valid, at the same time we must realize that a system of moral values in harmony with mammalian biology and therefore with human nature would have greater, not lesser, credibility. Such an ethical system would not only have a semblance of universality, it would also be more firmly rooted in the physical reality with which we must contend. The facts of nature do not necessarily supply us with what we should value, but if we can reasonably derive humane and beneficent considerations from the facts of nature and avoid the idiosyncrasies of reason unsupported by hard facts, why not lean in that direction?

This approach is consonant with Edward O. Wilson's statement that the study of natural selection "must be pursued to explain ethics."[6] Peter Singer, unlike many philosophers, accepts the influence of biology upon our ethical stance, but tends to use the biological aspect of altruism as the framework for ethics. He suggests that "our present ethical systems have their roots in the altruistic behavior of our early human and pre-human ancestors"[7] and that sociobiology "enables us to see ethics as a mode of human reasoning that develops in a group context, building on more limited, biologically based forms of altruism."[8]

Unlike Wilson and Singer, who suggest altruism and kinship as points of departure for the formation of an ethical system, I shall use the concept of harm avoidance as my frame of reference. It is a much more powerful force than the biological forces underlying kinship and altruism. But regardless which inherited behavior pattern we may use, Singer acknowledges that "we must return to biology to use our knowledge of human nature as a guide to what will or will not work as a code of ethics for normal human beings."[9]

Moral behavior is the product of our genetic imprints modified by human reason and emotion, as influenced by our physical and cultural environment. Our apparent ability to discipline and control our basic biological drives and constraints does not mean that they are an insignificant force underlying our behavior. The animalistic nature of humans may be hidden, but not ignored.

John Bowlby expressed this very strongly:

Those who dispute the view that there is in man behavior homologous with what in other species is traditionally called instinctive, have a heavy onus of proof on their hands. In respect to man's anatomical and physiological equipment a continuity in structure with that of other species is unquestionable. In respect to his behavioral equipment continuity of structure may be less evident, but were continuity to be totally absent all we know of man's evolution would be contradicted. What is far more probable than absence of continuity is, therefore, that the basic structure of man's behavioral equipment resembles that of infra-human species. . . . The early form is not superseded; it is modified, elaborated, and augmented but it still determines the overall pattern.[10]

We should assume that the laws of nature are morally neutral. It is in the human application of these laws that moral issues arise.

Within the diverse cultures of the world and despite their extremely broad spectrum of values, there are universal desires and behavior patterns, which reflect our biological inheritance. These human patterns are best seen, untrammeled by culture, in subhuman mammals.

Within the ecological constraints of nature mammals act aggressively to satiate hunger, procreate, feed and protect their young, gain power, and establish spheres of influence—patterns directed toward preservation of the self and preservation of the species.[11] Restraints that would prevent their freedom to act are resisted.

There is a unique relationship between these behavior patterns and the factor of harm. Regardless of their intensity, any and all desires are immediately negated when there is an imminent and unexpected threat of danger. Animals flee from harm and act forcefully to prevent it. The sudden threat of harm overwhelms and abolishes other feelings. This is a universal pattern in subhuman mammals and holds true for humans as well. The unique power of imminent danger to erase preexisting feelings suggests that the avoidance of harm is the most easily arousable biological reaction. It reflects the force of self-preservation impulses and is consistent with our understanding of emotion as described by James Papez and Paul MacLean.[12] I shall refer to this as the harm-avoidance factor. If we accept this understanding as valid it immediately becomes apparent that self-interest as reflected in the desire to avoid harm is biologically a preeminent force.[13]

What is the relationship between morality and the concept of harm-avoidance? First, what is harm?

Harm is ubiquitous and remains a possibility in every human relationship. It exists whenever an act is considered unacceptable by the individual acted upon. Unacceptable risk, imposition, deception, physical or mental pain are all forms of harm. Pain as an expected or possibly expected result of surgery or medical treatment, properly performed and with informed consent, is undesirable and hurtful, but cannot be considered harm since it is part of an acceptable risk. Harm involves an element of responsibility. Harm exists even if it is unknown to the person acted upon, such as revealing confidences obtained during the patient-doctor relationship, or not informing a patient of a mistake made during surgery that may affect the patient's future life. It is irrelevant whether the person is aware or unaware of the act, or even if it is impossible ever to be aware of the act, as with one who is deceased. Disrespect of the intent of the deceased constitutes harm.

The intent of the person who produces harm is not necessarily pertinent. Unintentional injury through accident is harm since it is without consent. It is the judgment of the person acted upon that determines whether harm does or does not exist.

Although many people may risk their lives for a cause, there does not appear to be any society or any individual who willingly accepts harm. If one accepts what is usually construed as, or what appears to be, harm, it is no longer harm but discomfort, pain, or even death for real or imagined gain. The martyr and the masochist fall into this niche.

In the balance of one person's rights against another person's desires, harm is to be expected. It is in the understanding of harm and the balancing of relative harms that the extent of freedoms can be delineated. It is in the values given the many types and degrees of harm that a balance can be reached between freedom to act and the harm that may be produced.

Since the desire to avoid harm is such a basic, intense and universal human attribute, its corollary, "do no harm," may be considered the most important rule to guide human behavior and therefore a primary moral principle. Where does the concept of harm-avoidance lead us?

Inherent in the universal desire to be free from harm is the desire to be free to act without restraint, for to restrain without consent is to commit harm. Since the principle must apply to all members of society and since unlimited freedom to act could be used to produce harm to others, freedom from harm and absolute freedom are incompatible as a social doctrine. Compromise is necessary. The essence of this compromise is that *individual freedom is inviolate as long as others are not harmed in the exercise of that freedom.* This suggests that autonomy, as qualified by nonmaleficence, may be considered the second ethical factor.

The influence of the harm-avoidance concept does not seem to stop there. Its significance becomes more apparent when we realize that every society, regardless of size or complexity, is a gregarious entity in which all members are to varying degrees interdependent. This is a biologically imposed constraint. As gregarious beings we cannot function adequately in an isolated mode. Without communal support to help obtain food and protection life would be endangered. Cooperation and compromise are necessary for humans to live together in relative harmony and for the protection of each and all and therefore for the "common good."

When we appreciate that the constraint of our gregarious nature forces a dependency of each upon the other to avoid harm, we are forced to realize that duties and obligations for the common good are, at the most fundamental level, harm-avoidance mechanisms. Working together for the common good enhances the survival of each individual as well as the group.

The universal need to consider the "common good," and its reciprocal duties and obligations between the community and the individual suggest that it may be reasonably considered the third ethical factor.

This raises several issues. How necessary for the welfare of society are the numerous demands of society? Where do we draw the line between what is necessary and what is simply desirable for physical comfort or psychological security? How do we evaluate the relative importance of a proposal for the "common good" in respect to its abridgement of an individual's freedom of choice? How should each person share in support of health, education, and other public services? These questions expose the conflict between individual "rights" and societal "needs and desires." This conflict as well as conflicts between individuals, again brings us to the essence of ethical problems, *the balancing of relative harms.*

Ethics is usually applied to relations between individuals, or between the individual and society, but within the relationship between the individual and society actions involving self assume ethical significance. This is especially pertinent to the physician. With the obligation and duty to act for the common good, lies the obligation to improve oneself, to nourish one's own talents. The more learned and skilled physicians become, the more valuable an asset they may be, both to themselves directly and to society, and thereby also indirectly to themselves. In a reciprocal manner there is a duty of society to enhance each citizen's ability to flourish. This reciprocity, along with the realization that society is composed of individuals, makes it reasonable to assume that each individual has some form of claim upon every other individual as well as on society as a whole. This issue involves the broad question of human and property rights. An extremely liberal and compassionate view of human rights is expressed by Henry Shue.[14]

Unfortunately there is no easy answer regarding how we are to balance general societal desires against individual autonomy, but the hierarchy within these values, which will be discussed later in this chapter, may serve as a guide.

As we continue to study the universal desire to avoid harm we expose an impetus toward beneficence. Although harm avoidance and beneficence may appear unrelated, harm avoidance serves as an underlying seed in the formation of beneficence. Beneficence and the common good are in many ways intertwined, but for the sake of clarity they will be considered as independent entities.

Beneficence may be defined as an action taken toward another person that is good for that person. It is the arm of benevolence, the desire to do good, but the intention underlying an act of beneficence may not necessarily reflect benevolence. One may be forced to do an act of goodness unwillingly, or do it for purely selfish reasons.

There are five biologically influenced elements that serve as the seed underlying the formation of beneficence. Three are basically harm-avoidance mechanisms. The fourth is related to altruism and the fifth is related to the concept of mastery.

Notwithstanding occasional bizarre exceptions, humans tend to form an intense bond to progeny. We develop an unquestionable inclination to protect, feed, guard, and love our offspring. As a result of our desire to protect our offspring we hope that others will act beneficently toward them. We also hope, as a result of personal insecurity that, if necessary, society will deal kindly with us. This leads to the realization that for reciprocity to take place each person should act beneficently toward others. To help insure one's own security, social patterns to foster such attitudes are encouraged. Although this psychodynamic is rarely part of our consciousness during an act of beneficence, we are nevertheless unconsciously inclined, at least to some extent, to accept the obligation of beneficence not simply because we are so nice, but because beneficence within the social group is a protective device that may prevent hurt to ourselves and our young.

The second harm-avoidance factor that helps in the

formation of societal beneficence is possibly of minimal significance, but warrants mentioning. Biologically, there is no compelling reason to prevent parents from stealing or killing in order to feed a child if food cannot be obtained otherwise. In almost all human societies, past and present, there are usually a few who have much and many who have little. The potential threat of force by those whose "little" becomes insufficient to support life, especially in the presence of affluence, is very real. It therefore behooves societies, if only from the point of self-interest, to assist those in need in order to avert social strife in the future as the population continues to explode and poverty and hunger persists.

The same condition of poverty elicits the third harm-avoidance factor that supports beneficence. It is a psychological element, which is minimally, if at all, biologically driven. It is related to the anguish and guilt of those who live in comfort when made aware of the prevalence and anguish of hunger. Within the act of beneficence that helps to diminish the agony of those in need, lies the avoidance of the guilt we may feel for not helping, or not helping them as much as we could.[15] Philanthropy not only serves society, but secondarily diminishes this form of harm to the self.

The fourth element is reflected in a pattern of behaviors resembling beneficence frequently observed among many gregarious mammals, despite certain exceptions such as male polar bears killing cubs. These include adoption of orphans among the primates, none of which involves the close bond of parents and offspring,[16] and the danger-alerting signals of the gazelle. This seemingly altruistic and kinship-related behavior does not imply the feeling of altruism as we know it in humans, although the behavior pattern appears similar to what would be considered beneficence in people. Although one cannot prove this thesis, this protective species-preservation mechanism is probably part of the human genetic makeup.

The fifth element is inherent in the feeling of benevolence, and in the act of beneficence. It is the psychodynamic that produces pleasure, conscious or unconscious, that is derived from the organically based sense of mastery[17] associated with acts of altruism. It is an ever-present and subtle factor in philanthropy.

It is a strange paradox that elements in human nature such as self-centeredness, insecurity, fear, and the desire for mastery, which may produce unkind and harmful acts toward others, also serve as subtle factors supporting the formation of human beneficence. In spite of this duality, the fact that they contribute to the formation of humane qualities tends to negate the concern, often expressed by creationists, that Darwinism "seemed to threaten the foundation of public morality."[18]

Although the above organic and societal aspects serve as the seed in the formation of beneficence, they only account for a small part in its overall development. Its development is markedly enhanced by secular and religious philosophies that expound love and kindness.

Throughout the world's religious literature, the element of benevolence is impressed upon us in the commands to "love thy neighbor as thyself," and "do to others as you would have others do to you." The behavior required by the application of these concepts is not a pattern in nature. They are, as Thomas Hobbes expresses it, "contrary to our natural passions,"[19] but their presence has a pervasive effect upon the minds of people. Without our awareness of such concepts and traditions and our feeble attempts to live according to them, our lives would be colder, more detached, and less humane.

There is one aspect of beneficence that must be approached cautiously. Since we are morally obligated, under the factors of common good and beneficence, to help those in need, society may rightfully hold that a person should be held legally as well as morally responsible for hurt done as a result of inaction. This would be difficult to legislate because it is so difficult to delineate all the possible variations of human interaction. Think of the near-infinite gradations to be drawn between the two extremes of, on the one hand, condemning a person who does not wish to risk his or her life to save a child who has just fallen through thin ice, and, on the other hand, refusing to soothe a person frightened by lightning? The impossibility of demarcating the relative importance of each facet of the situation and penetrating the thoughts of a bystander suggests that inaction leading to someone's hurt must be judged with great forbearance. Mill appreciated the danger of this stand and stated that such a decision "requires a much more cautious exercise of compulsion."[20]

In spite of the difficulty of evaluating a bystander's thoughts, moral criticism regarding inaction is probably warranted if it is confined to three specific limits. First, there is no doubt that the bystander is fully aware of the harmful or potentially harmful situation. Second, the bystander need not place him- or herself in significant danger, however one measures significant. Third, the effort necessary to help is not beyond reasonable limits. Defining what is considered harmful, serious, dangerous, or reasonable is always problematic, but this is a constant in every moral decision and one that we must live with. This dilemma has been well described by Marc Franklin in his discussion of The Good Samaritan Law which obligates people to help one in distress.[21]

THE HIERARCHY WITHIN THE FOUR FACTORS

In the derivation of nonmaleficence and freedom it is apparent that freedom is slightly in a secondary position since it is derived from and modified by the factor of nonmaleficence.

As far as "common good" and beneficence are concerned, the pattern of behavior in subhuman mammals,
and which has been carried forward into all human cultures, suggests that concern for both of these factors is,
except for family relationships, quite subservient to a person's desire to be unharmed and free to act. Each individual is inclined to act as a self-centered unit, generally
beneficent to others only when it is comfortable to do so,
or when it serves the individual's self-interest materially
or psychologically. This is well described in Peter Singer's
book *The Expanding Circle.*[22]

Although it is not possible to establish precise priority
values for the four factors in numerical terms, the factors
of nonmaleficence and autonomy stand above both the
common good and beneficence, while the common good
stands significantly above beneficence. The basis of this
hierarchy is its biological reality. This does not mean that
the hierarchy is what should be, but only that it exists as
part of human genetic inheritance and is therefore consonant with human nature.

If we ignore biological influences and thereby under-
value the significance of harm avoidance as a powerful
common human attribute, then all four factors may be
considered as equal, or any one may be given preference.
On the other hand, if human nature is respected, then we
may more readily accept their position in the hierarchy of
values. This latter approach, which places nonmaleficence and individual freedom at a higher relative value
than the common good and beneficence, tends to support
a free society. The danger in this approach is that unbri-
dled respect for personal freedom may diminish one's
sense of obligation toward the common good and beneficence. But respect for nonmaleficence and individual freedom, even if held paramount, need not reduce our sense
of humanism and our thrust to do good. There is no doubt
that arrogance of autonomy can lead to social indiffer-

ence, but undue importance given the common good may lead to social tyranny. Overemphasis of the common good may assume extremely dangerous if not deadly aspects. Stalin's tragic program for the Soviet Union was not only to increase and secure his power base but also conceived as best for the common good of that nation. To diminish the importance of nonmaleficence and autonomy is to invite imprisonment of our minds if not our bodies. The danger of the misuse of an excess of autonomy within the constraint of nonmaleficence is small compared to the danger of misuse of the common-good factor if made supreme in the decision-making process. Both approaches are double-edged swords, but safety lies in that approach which is more closely in tune with human nature.

There is a wide spectrum between those who approach a situation without any clear-cut rules upon which to base a decision except what the individual feels is best and those who accept rules that must be followed regardless of consequences. I believe it is important to accept a more central position and to consider the four moral factors as relatively firmly based, deontological concepts, which should be balanced in each situation. If we do not, we will be inclined to change our moral frame of reference as circumstances vary. To enter a situation without precise, firmly grounded moral precepts and respect for the hierarchy between them, suggests that whenever we navigate the stormy sea of decision-making, we can jump from one ethical boat to another if it appears more convenient or safe.

The fear that firmly grounded moral principles will not meet changing times does not appear to be valid. Changing circumstances do not require new ethical values in order to be dealt with properly. Changing circumstances demand only an understanding of basic principles and the ability to properly extrapolate those principles to a new situation. Within the concept of "balancing" the pertinent moral factors lies the needed flexibility. An obvious example of this type of balance is the weighing of relative harms underlying a good lie. It is necessary at times to lie to a suicide-prone patient who is faced with news of a tragic disease. Such a "white lie" causes much less harm than the potential harm to that person if the truth were told.

There are no clear-cut rules as to how to apply these factors to a given situation. What is crucial is to develop the attitude that respects their hierarchical relationship. This respect, and the understanding that balancing the ethical equation is essentially measuring the relative harms and gains that may result, should be a helpful guide. Even though the hierarchy may be rightfully over-turned, depending upon the balance of relative values and harms, it would be unfortunate to ignore it in any attempt to solve an ethical problem.

It is not mere coincidence that the four moral factors derived from harm-avoidance are consonant with religious and humanistic concepts of human morality. The common interest to consider the avoidance of harm as a basis for the development of good human behavior has been expressed as a single dictum for more than two millennia as the negatively stated form of the Golden Rule, "Do not to others what you would not have others do to you." It was expressed in Hinduism,[23] Confucianism,[24] Buddhism,[25] Zoroastrianism,[26] and Judaism.[27] Although the axiom is not expressed as such, the essence of the concept is also within Islamic theology. The same maxim was part of Christianity during the early centuries. It was also expressed in ancient times outside of a religious context by Philo and Isocrates.[28] This single concept has been and probably still is the most universally accepted summary underlying the principles of human conduct.

This maxim forces us to ask what we would not have others do to ourselves. It appears at first to be simply a restraining concept, directed toward satisfying the common desire of all people to be free of harm. But it is obviously more than a restraining concept. It is not simply coincidence that this maxim is essentially identical to the universal human attribute from which the four moral factors have been derived. There appears to be exquisite wisdom in this negative maxim. Although love and benevolence are not ordered, beneficence is. Through understanding and living the ramifications of this single concept people and societies could live without conflict.

The supportive directive "love thy neighbor" and the positive form of the Golden Rule, expressed by Jainism as ". . . he should . . . treat all beings as he himself would be treated"[29] and later by Jesus, served to emphasize the obligation to do good inherent in the negatively stated rule. They stressed the need to feel concern for and kindness to others, to act with tenderness and compassion, and to feel that sense of mutual concern that is the hallmark of a truly humane society. This humane social consciousness has permeated human thinking in spite of the hate, bigotry, intolerance, and war that have marked our path.

The combination of these two thoughts are probably more crucial to the physician than to any other professional. The single most important concept impressed upon every medical student is to "Do No Harm." Soon after that the student is exposed to the need to feel and express compassion, to take the time to touch and ease the heartache of his or her patient. One may not reach the point of loving his or her neighbor, but tender, loving care comes close to it.

However, we must not assume that what is admirable is synonymous with what is morally mandatory. This difference exposes an important parameter of secular ethics. An act that may be admirable and may enhance our lives and the lives of others may be beyond the demands of morality. The constraints surrounding beneficence, as previously described, force this conclusion. To "love your neighbor" is magnificent and to forgive a thief or even a murderer is magnanimous. Such actions add a quality of graciousness and nobility to life, but to assume that such admirable traits are mandated by ethics would be unwarranted.

Now the important question: Why should these four factors be accepted as the elements that need to be balanced when evaluating an ethical problem rather than another set of factors derived from a different frame of reference?

There are five reasons: (1) they are consonant with a universal pattern of human behavior; (2) they are consonant with biological forces and therefore consonant with human nature; (3) they are not derived from any single national, cultural, or religious format; (4) they do not make impossible or unreasonable demands upon people; and (5) they are consonant with the most common religious and secular tenet enunciated to guide human behavior.

The question arises as to whether specific criteria may be stated for properly balancing the moral factors. This does not appear feasible, but the following thoughts may at least partially speak to this problem.

Any moral principle may be misused. The four moral factors—nonmaleficence, autonomy, common good, and beneficence—comprise an equation that must be balanced within the constraint of prudence in order to determine whether a particular action is ethical or not. Prudence is mandated by this approach to ethics. It is the protector of self-interest inherent within the idea of harm-avoidance.

I would like to stress that I am not thinking in terms of rules of morality but rather of four factors that when properly balanced by "dispassionate" reason as applied to a given situation should result in a decision that is more likely to be morally correct. It is necessary to realize that none of the factors can stand as isolated moral axioms and that the hierarchical relationship between them must be appreciated.

The general approach in the evaluation of an ethical problem would be to use the classical role-reversal test: identify all elements in the situation; evaluate their significance; decide which of the moral factors are applicable, keeping in mind the hierarchy among the factors; psychologically place yourself on both sides of the issue; ask what you would not wish done to yourself; and then, if harm is an inevitable byproduct of the situation, make decisions that minimize the harm. I would like to stress that I am expressing a negative concept. *What is pertinent is not what we would want, but rather what we would not want.*

In the process of making decisions regarding a patient's health, this general approach to ethics becomes crucial, especially the concept of putting yourself into the patient's position. It is not without good reason that patients often ask a surgeon, "Would you operate if your child or spouse were the patient?" Unfortunately doctors do not always place themselves on the opposite side of the fence when a decision is made regarding the value of surgery or medical treatment.

NOTES

1. Ethics is derived from the Greek *ethikos* which pertains to customs and manners. Ethikos was probably translated into Latin by Cicero as *moralis,* using the word *mores* as the base, which pertains to customs and manners.

2. William K. Frankena, *Ethics,* 2nd ed., Foundation of Philosophy Series (Englewood Cliffs, N.J.: Prentice-Hall Inc., 1973), p. 8.

3. Immanuel Kant utilized the approach of reason and established his now famous "categorical imperative" stating that "I ought never to act except in such a way that I can also will that my maxim should become a universal law." Immanuel Kant, *Groundwork of the Metaphysic of Morals,* trans. H. J. Paton (New York: Harper and Row, 1964), p.70. Several secondary formulations of the imperative were expressed to help

clarify his intent. Terry Nardin succinctly clarifies its function. "The categorical imperative is not itself a rule of conduct but a criterion or test of the moral validity of particular rules." Terry Nardin, *Law, Morality and the Relations of States* (Princeton: Princeton University Press, 1983), p. 231. Kant's imperative would serve well as an evaluator of moral rules when used within a given society, but a rule that would satisfy that society would not necessarily be acceptable in a different culture.

4. Thomas Donaldson, "Kant's Global Rationalism," in *Traditions of International Ethics,* edited by Terry Nardin and David Maple (Cambridge: Cambridge University Press, 1992), p. 141.

5. Peter Singer, *The Expanding Circle* (New York: Farrar, Straus and Giroux 1981), p. 53.

6. Edward O. Wilson, *Sociobiology: The Abridged Version* (Cambridge: Belknap Press of Harvard University Press, 1980), p. 3.

7. Singer, *The Expanding Circle,* p. 5.

8. Ibid., p. 149.

9. Ibid., p. 158.

10. John Bowlby, *Attachment and Loss,* vol.1 (New York: Basic Books, 1969), p. 40.

11. James W. Papez, "A Proposed Mechanism of Emotion," *Archives of Neurology And Psychiatry* 38 (1937): 725–43. Paul D. MacLean, "The Limbic System with Respect to Self-Preservation and the Preservation of the Species," *Journal of Nervous and Mental Diseases* 127 (1958): 22.

12. Papez, "A Proposed Mechanism of Emotion," pp. 1–11.

13. This is consonant with Hobbes's belief that man's relationship to society is one of self-interest, but there is a major difference between where this concept leads Hobbes and where I move with it. Thomas Hobbes, *Man and Citizen (De Homine and De Cive),* edited by Bernard Gert (Indianapolis: Hackett Publishing Company, 1993), *De Cive,* chap. 1, #2, p. 115.

14. Henry Shue, *Basic Rights: Subsistence, Affluence, and U.S. Foreign Policy* (Princeton: Princeton University Press, 1980). R. J. Vincent has written an excellent short discussion of human rights as it relates to international affairs: "The Idea of Rights in International Ethics," in *International Ethics,* edited by Terry Nardin and David Mapel (Cambridge: Cambridge University Press, 1992), pp. 250–66. See Appendix F. regarding human and property rights.

15. Concept suggested by Richard J. Regan, personal communication, 1991.

16. Singer, *The Expanding Circle*, pp. 6–7.

17. See Appendix A: Discussion of Mastery.

18. Bernard I. Davis, "Novel Pressures on the Advance of Science," *Annals of the New York Academy of Sciences* 265 (1976): 204

19. Thomas Hobbes, *Leviathan* (New York: Bobbs-Merrill, 1958), p. 139.

20. John Stuart Mill, "On Liberty," in *Essential Works of John Stuart Mill*, edited by Max Lerner (New York: Bantam Matrix Edition, Bantam Books, 1965), p. 264.

21. Marc A. Franklin, "Vermont Requires Rescue, a Comment," *Stanford Law Review* 25 (1972): 51–61.

22. See note 5 for complete reference.

23. H. T. D. Rost, *The Golden Rule* (Oxford: George Ronald, 1986), p. 28.

24. Arthur Waley, trans., *The Analects of Confucius* (New York: Vintage Books, 1983), Book XII, #2, and Book XV 23, p. 198.

25. Rost, *The Golden Rule*, p. 40, Udana-Varga 5, 18.

26. Ibid., p. 57, Dadistan-I-Dinik 94:5

27. Edgar J. Goodspeed, trans., *Book of Tobit* (New York: Vintage Books, 1959), sect. 4, #15, p. 115. *Talmud Bavli— Babylonian Talmud* (Jerusalem: Israel Institute for Talmud Publications, 1968), vol. II, Shah. 31, ARN 15, 61, pp. 126–27.

28. James Hastings, ed., *Encyclopedia of Religion and Ethics* (New York: Charles Scribner's Sons, 1914), vol. 6, p. 311.

29. *Sutrakritanka*, Book 1, Lecture 10, in *The Sacred Books of the East*, edited by F. Max Müller (Delhi: Motilal Banarsidass 1989), vol. 45, p. 307.

2

General Problems in Application

There are a number of problems which arise when society attempts to introduce any ethical format into its structure. Two of these problems concern the principal of beneficence and the psychological implication of law.

THE PROBLEM OF OVERPROTECTION

Beneficence can be overdone by overzealous segments of society. It may be applied to someone who does not wish to be helped. This raises several questions: When should beneficence be invoked in a complex society? Are good motivations always the best indicators of right or wrong? Where do we draw the line that balances our sense of concern and benevolence against an individual's freedom of choice? Does the "good" imposed justify the negation of personal freedom?

Beneficence becomes dangerous when it is imposed on a competent person. There is a tendency for many well-meaning but self-righteous individuals to impose their values upon others who are fully competent but who have a different sense of values. John Stuart Mill wrote forcefully about the problem of unrequested and unwarranted beneficence:

His own good, either physical or moral, is not a sufficient warrant. He cannot rightfully be compelled to do or forbear because it will be better for him to do so, because it would make him happier, because, in the opinion of others, to do so would be wise, or even right. . . . Over himself, over his own body and mind, the individual is sovereign.[1]

Because of the danger posed by unrequested beneficence, in law it has only been imposed upon those who were considered incompetent, namely on children because of their immaturity or adults on the basis of mental disturbance. This raises the question of what we mean by "competence."

DETERMINING COMPETENCE

The determination of competency is a problem without clean-cut lines of demarcation. Without precise guidelines incompetence regarding children has been determined according to the designated age when the child is generally considered mature enough to make proper judgments with respect to his or her welfare. This is obviously an arbitrary determination, but one reference point has been the age when someone may be conscripted to fight in defense of the nation. Clearly this age varies with each country.

In regard to the adult, any individual considered competent to write a last will and testament may be considered intellectually and emotionally competent to make any life decision. Competence assumes that the individual can understand the pertinent facts and issues in question, reasonably and rationally evaluate the data, and understand the consequences of a decision. All of these requirements are subjective. What is reasonable? How much understanding exists? How rational is rational? There are no tests to assess these variables accurately. There is a very grey area between what would constitute legal incompetence and relative inability to make a decision. Therefore, when competency is questioned, except in urgent medical situations when the opinion of one or more physicians may suffice, it should be resolved at a judicial hearing, after due process, in order to protect the individual's autonomy.

But in real-life situations, although competence is essentially a legal concept, physicians must still evaluate the ability of the patient to understand, and to make an informed decision, in order to feel secure that the patient truly has given "informed consent" to start or continue medical treatment. Physicians therefore work within Sidney Wanzer's phrase "decision-making capacity,"[2] since they do not have the right legally to use the word *competence* when determining the patient's ability to understand. For physicians to do so places them in jeopardy. To a certain degree this may be a legal loophole. It is not pragmatically possible to seek legal recourse in every borderline case. Therefore, the "decision-making capacity" may not always be synonymous with competency from the legal point of view since the physician and family may be less rigid in their evaluation of a patient's ability to make a medical decision. Adequate or inadequate decision-making capacity is, in practice, almost always determined by the physician in conjunction with the family if there is any doubt. Other health-care personnel are rarely involved in this decision. Adequate decision-making capacity, like competency, demands that the patient must not only be free to make a choice but understand the risks and benefits of any decision, in other words, the patient must appreciate the significance of the most important variables pertinent to the situation. The only real difference between "decision-making capacity" and "competence" lies in who makes the evaluation.

Because of the danger of infringing upon individual rights through the misuse of the concept of incompetence, the courts have become very cautious about declaring someone to be incompetent. As a result several principles have been established in our society.

(A) Incompetence generally refers to the inability of persons to manage their own affairs or to understand the issues in question and the consequences of their decisions.

(B) Incompetence generally applies to children (between arbitrary chronological age limits), the mentally ill, the senile, or the comatose.

(C) All adults are competent to make personal decisions until proven otherwise as determined through judicial due process.

(D) A decision made while competent is not to be ignored simply because the individual who made the decision becomes incompetent at a later date. If so, all wills could be ignored.

(E) Incompetence is limited to the specific inabilities involved; therefore, incompetence in one area does not imply total incompetence. There are gradations of incompetence.

The restriction of imposing beneficence only upon the incompetent person reflects society's high respect for the importance of individual freedom of choice and an awareness of the danger of unrequested beneficence. In essence, beneficence should be invoked only with the consent of the recipient if competent, or if we assume the incompetent person would consent if competent.

A PSYCHOLOGICAL IMPLICATION OF LAW

The fact that a law or regulation exists creates a potentially undesirable illusion. Its mere presence suggests that it is right and just. Law molds public thought. Permission gained through law is frequently thought of, and accepted, as a fundamental ethical right rather than simply the granting by society of a legal right.

We are dealing with a potential Pandora's box centered around the word *rights*. For in the minds of the public, a *legal* right becomes a *basic* right. This extrapolation is then used as a basis to gain other similar "rights." Because society grants a student the right to be educated through high school without tuition does not imply that the student has the right to additional educational support through college and professional school. Certainly students have the right to ask society for such support. If it is given, it would reflect society's belief that further education would be of benefit to all of society and therefore supported by the pillar of common good. But it is not a student's right because of a legal right to partial education. There is a fundamental right to seek education, but not a right to education of any form at any time. This distinction between the *right to seek* and the *right to have* what one desires is often confused in modern times.

The development of such psychological trends tends to erode individual rights under the guise of serving the common good. This is suggested by Joseph Fletcher's statement that "as needs change with changing conditions so rights should change too. . . . It is human needs that validate rights, not the other way around."[3]

Henry Veatch appears to agree with Fletcher's concept of new rights arising out of social change. He offers this suggestion:

> Until this century health care could be treated as a luxury, no matter how offensive this might be now. The amount of real healing that went on was minimal anyway. But now, with the biological revolution, health care really is essential to "life, liberty and the pursuit of happiness," and health care is a right for everyone because of the social revolution, which is really a revolution in our conception of justice.[4]

This concept is difficult to accept unless it is understood to mean only a legal right and not a fundamental right, otherwise fundamental rights now become life, liberty, medical care, and the pursuit of happiness. Why not legal care and shelter as well? Within the statement, "It is human needs that validate rights," lies a concept that is much too dependent upon fashion and one's definition of "need." Each and every citizen must have access to health care. The thrust, the drive, to provide this service should be no less intense simply because it is based upon society's obligation, under the factors of common good and beneficence, than it would be if based upon the concept of an ethical right to health care. Laws should be passed that would supply medical care to those who need it. But the ethical right regarding health care is only the right to *seek* it.

This concept of "right" is obviously not consonant with biology. It is expected, normal, and natural for a starving animal to take what food it needs to survive, even at the point of cannibalism. But in a human social framework, if we expand needs to the status of fundamental rights, we open a Pandora's box. The need of the starving must be recognized and alleviated by society not because a fundamental right is being ignored but because the common good and beneficence demands that starvation be eliminated.

NOTES

1. Max Lerner, ed., *Essential Works of John Stuart Mill* (New York: Bantam Matrix Edition, Bantam Books, 1965), p. 263.

2. Sidney H. Wanzer et al., "The Physician's Responsibility Toward Hopelessly Ill Patients," *New England Journal of Medicine* 320, no. 13 (March 30, 1989): 845.

3. Joseph Fletcher, "Ethical Aspects of Genetic Control," *New England Journal of Medicine* 258 (1971): 776-83, p. 782.

4. Robert Veatch, "Models for Ethical Medicine in a Revolutionary Age," *Hastings Center Report* 2, no. 3 (June 1971): 5.

3

The Doctor-Patient Relationship

People seeking medical care are concerned with the most vital aspects of their existence: health and life. Yet their traditional role in this relationship has been remarkably passive. The amazing absence of questioning or challenge to physicians is rarely seen in any other consumer-supplier relationship. It reflects the respect and confidence that has been traditionally granted physicians and this professional group's unique body of knowledge.

The patients' attitudes toward their physicians are usually ones of trust. Those who are ill believe physicians are dedicated to the welfare of their patients and will act to the best of their professional ability. This is in part due to an awareness that the motivation, training, and discipline of medical students is directed toward helping those who are ill. Medical students soon become aware of this sense of trust, not only by the readiness of patients to expose the nakedness of their bodies for examination, but often to expose their innermost private thoughts unrelated to their physical problems. The significance and importance of this intimate relationship is constantly stressed during the students' training. It is an important factor in the formation of the doctor's paternalistic attitude. This human relationship, from the physicians' point of view, is one of the most gratifying aspects of the practice of medicine, but at times it can also be overwhelming.

Patients expect physicians to be more than repositories of facts. The hope is that physicians will have the ability to sense in another human the significance, both personal and social, of anguish of many types and degrees and will be open and responsive to patients' doubts and apprehensions. The expected response from the physician to this trust and hope is dedication, integrity, and respect of confidences—the foundation of the traditional covenant between doctor and patient.

The physician's sensitivity to the emotional needs of the patient are, or should be, almost as important as technical skill and judgment. The totality of the patient is in need when any aspect of that patient is in need. It is the touch and the gentle word that is sometimes more potent than the antibiotic or knife. Unfortunately this is not always seen in practice.

Human potential is so immense that the psychic drive toward health, if harnessed, may be as therapeutic as any drug. Because the psychological aspect of health is so pertinent to physical health, the tendency to avoid answering bothersome phone calls—to insert martinet secretaries as buffers between patient and doctor and to blur the responsibility as to whom the family and patient may call to discuss problems during a complicated team treatment program—should be avoided.

Within this framework of trust, patients develop faith in the doctors' knowledge and integrity. This trust is not so much in the ability of the physicians as it is in the doctors' honesty. The patients have faith that physicians will not attempt that which is beyond their ability and will seek consultation if necessary. This confidence permits a mother or father to allow a neurosurgeon, a person they have just met, to enter into the brain of their child and operate in an area where life and death are intertwined, with confidence that the surgeon will act toward that child with the same care as if the child were the doctor's own.

This traditional tie between doctor and patient has a unique character that exists nowhere else in the human experience. Its remarkable quality lies in the strength of the empathy that develops between them and the amazing speed of its formation. But this highly personal relationship has been deteriorating in recent years. There are many reasons for this. The paternalistic attitude of the physician carries within it an undesirable element, one that is sometimes translated into a style of autocracy ("Just do as I say, I know what is best for you"). On other occasions the covenant, the dedication to help all aspects of patient needs, has at times been misused. There has been a tendency to blot out patients' overt or hidden doubts ("You don't really need a consultation, I have no doubt about the treatment program") and not to alert patients fully to alternatives, let alone referring the patient to a more experienced and superior surgeon. It is common for physicians to make great effort to identify the better doctor to treat their families, but to not question their ability to treat their own patients. In addition, many physicians have been unwilling to take the time to explain problems to patients, or to share the responsibility of decision making with the patient, especially in view of the increasing complexity of medical science. This was based on a usually mistaken belief that the patient may not understand the problem, or could not bear "bad news." It is true that, occasionally, patients would signal that they didn't really want to know, and some patients are simply not capable of understanding the situation, but generally it is remarkable how well patients comprehend complex problems if given time to understand.

Although historically these decisions were the private domain of the physician, contemporary society is now inclined to reject this kind of paternalism. Patients now want to have a better understanding of their illness and a more active role in deciding the course of their treatment. This demand, as opposed to mere acceptance of a doctor's recommendations, reflects a diminished element of faith in the physician, and it is understandable. To allow someone to affect and invade one's life is frightening. Other reasons for patient skepticism include the overwhelming expense of illness, the difficulty of having one's physician readily available, the apparent callousness of some physicians and the occasional exposure to a dishonest or incompetent doctor. One of the byproducts is the development of a litigious society. A new concept, "defensive medicine," is now part of the consciousness of doctors.

The individual's desire for a more active role in the decision-making process has contributed to an obvious change in the doctor-patient relationship. It has lost much of its symbolic covenant nature and has become more of a contractual agreement with all of its legalistic implications.[1] This has both good and bad features. An important and good aspect of this change is the reduction of physician autocracy and a recognition of patients' dignity and right to control their own lives.

The responsibility and empathy of a covenant relationship were readily accepted by physicians when they saw themselves in a parental role, but this has changed, especially since the public has become more knowledgeable, less passive, and much more litigious. The covenant was broad and trusting; the contract is narrow and exacting.

For physicians the covenant is not as protective as a contract. This danger is reflected in the *Mohr* v. *Williams* case.[2] Dr. Williams had consent to operate on the patient's right ear. But after the patient was anesthetized Williams discovered that the left ear was in greater need of surgery than the right. He therefore treated the left ear. It was quite apparent that the patient would have permitted the surgery if he had been informed of the condition of the left ear prior to being anesthetized. Medically and ethically the surgeon was correct, yet legally he was at fault and was found guilty of battery. The covenant was not broken, but the contract was. It is because of such cases that physicians and surgeons are now inclined to practice "defensive" medicine. They must think in terms of contracts rather than covenants. If this is done too literally it works to the detriment of both parties.

It would be extremely unfortunate if as a result of the contract concept the sense of paternalism toward the patient were lost. Although a contract may interfere in the covenant relationship, there is a duty to respect the healing power in the quality of trust in the covenant relationship. It is the covenant relationship, not the contract, that drives the physician to go that extra mile. This force as well as the healing power should not be lost in the development of a contract. Never in the contractual relationship should there be an absence of the sense of compassion and dedication inherent within the covenant. It is within the covenant relationship, not the contract, that patients feel secure and sheltered. The obligation of the physician is to continue *to act in the manner of a gentle parental figure* to foster this feeling. This is not simply due to a desire to fulfill the factor of beneficence but is in actuality the doctor's function; it is his or her charge as a physician. In this regard, if a patient were to refuse therapy necessary for health, the physician must not simply acquiesce, which would be the easy thing to do and would be acceptable within the contract concept, but must bring forth the strongest influence short of coercion to change the patient's mind, as a covenant would demand.

In a discussion of the covenant-contract relationship, Dr. Lynn Peterson[3] of Harvard Medical School described a case that revealed a possible advantage for the patient within the contract state. He described the case of a young man who underwent an abdominal operation for appendicitis. During surgery it was apparent that the actual problem was one involving part of the colon, the sigmoid. In the judgment of the surgeon a resection of the sigmoid, with temporary placement of the colon opening through the wall of the abdomen (a colostomy), would be the procedure of choice since, in his opinion, in this particular circumstance, to treat the condition without surgery carried a 70 percent probability that the patient would have to repeat the operation to resect the sigmoid. But since he had not discussed the possibility of a temporary colostomy and since there was a 30 percent chance of success with medical management, he closed the abdomen without performing the additional surgery that he would have done if he were only working within the framework of a covenant. On hindsight, when everyone is brilliant, the contract worked in favor of the patient since the conservative approach was successful. But also only the patient could know the value for him of that 30 percent chance of avoiding the surgery and its effects.

It is important at this juncture to clarify the principles that underlie the patient's rights and the physician's role in this new contractual relationship.

PATIENTS' RIGHTS

The privilege to treat patients is granted the physician by those who ask for care. The physician brings to the patient the knowledge of disease and the skill to treat it. The doctor thus becomes an agent of the patient. Neither the physician nor the patient must ever lose sight of that very simple fact. The physician may be in a position of action, but the patient wields the power. The patient always has the final right of decision.[4]

Patients have the right not to seek medical care as long as they are not suffering from a disease that may harm others if untreated, such as a contagious or infectious disease. They have the right to select the physician they desire; to discharge the physician; to cancel, refuse, and forbid medical care so long as harm to others is not a significant factor.

Patients have the right to be adequately informed in order to make a decision regarding their own care. This is the essence of informed consent. As Norman Cantor expresses it: "The doctrine of informed consent is grounded on the premise that a physician's judgment is subservient to the patient's right of self-determination."[5] Informed consent demands that physicians provide patients with enough data for a "reasonable" person to make a decision regarding therapy. This assumes that the most important and most common risks inherent in a properly performed procedure are presented to patients. Although each and every complication cannot be reasonably tabulated in complex situations, at least the most serious risks must be disclosed. That at least includes blindness, death, paralysis, deafness, sterility, impotence, and disfigurement.

The right to be adequately informed is based upon patients' freedom of choice, which becomes compromised if they are not given adequate data upon which to make judicious choices regarding the harm-benefit ratio of different treatments or lack of treatment. Informed consent also implies awareness of alternate treatment programs. In addition, it implies disclosure of any limitations of the facility in which the procedure may be done and adequate knowledge conveyed regarding special medical skills available elsewhere.

It must be considered an ethical imperative to adequately inform patients of all pertinent data in order to enable them to make decisions. This consent is to satisfy legal requirements, but the physician should regard the process of obtaining informed consent as important as, if not more important than, patients' signatures on essential forms. It is in the process of obtaining informed consent that a proper rapport is established with patients. To treat without consent is to commit battery. To avoid the issue of battery, consent—either oral, implied, or written—must be given. The courts have long supported this right of privacy. In the case of *Pratt* v. *Davis*, an Illinois appeals court held:

"Under a free government . . . the . . . citizen's . . . right . . . forbids a physician to violate without permission, the bodily integrity of his patient."[6]

The need to inform the patient of potential risks first arose in the case of *Natanson* v. *Kline*.[7] In this case a patient was told to undergo X-ray therapy and was not informed about the risks of radiation burn to the surrounding tissues. The court asserted that the physician must disclose the nature of the illness, the nature of the proposed treatments, the probability of success, the alternative treatment programs, the risks of unfortunate results, and unforeseen conditions. The usual basis for legal action against a physician under the concept of informed consent is the assumption that if the patient were fully informed of the risks of the procedure, the treatment would probably have been refused. The frame of reference for judgment is whether or not an average reasonable person would have accepted the treatment if aware of the possible complications.

Informed consent does not demand that physicians alert patients to the details of each and every medication prescribed unless it is generally considered a high-risk drug by the medical community. The acceptance of medication, without detailed explanation of the action of each drug, implies informed consent to receive treatment according to the physician's best judgment. It is within this parameter that placebos* may be given without any sense of a moral breach. Certainly, if a patient asks for specific details, the explanation must be forthcoming.

Placebo therapy is usually used to determine the actual need for strong analgesics. The use of placebos does not imply distrust or contempt for the patient. If the placebo proves to be efficacious, it does not necessarily mean that

---

*Medication given to test the psychological aspect of the complaint of pain. The patient is unaware that the pill or injection is not a standard painkiller.

the patient's request for analgesics is without basis. Placebos may act on both organic as well as psychological pain. The placebo itself, as it impinges upon the psyche, may increase the production of endorphins, substances the body produces that can reduce pain. It may be very important for patients to learn whether or not they are placebo responders. Its successful use, when explained to patients, may encourage them to more adequately exploit their own hidden power—the power of belief—of the optimistic smile. The physician takes a certain risk when using a placebo. Patients may not appreciate that this type of deception is in their best interests, or be willing to accept that their pain may have an emotional component, which may then be helped by better understanding the relationship between the psyche and pain. If a patient's reaction is one of anger, the doctor has not only lost a patient but may have his or her reputation unfairly sullied in the community. Angered patients are very prone to do so. As a result, some insecure physicians may use a placebo but refrain from revealing the data to the patient.

THE PHYSICIAN'S ROLE

Through centuries of custom and supported by the judiciary, certain rights have been retained by physicians. These include the right not to accept someone as a patient. (This formerly held true even in emergency situations, but there are some recent changes in law that may obligate any person to help in an emergency situation.[8]) Doctors have the right to resign from the management of a case, but once a physician accepts an ill person as his or her patient (and I very specifically use the possessive case*), the doctor cannot

---

*I use the possessive case, his/her, since the patient should be considered as part of the doctor's extended family. This is an integral part of covenant as opposed to the contract.

leave that patient unless arrangements have been made or can be made for some other physician to assume the responsibility of therapy. Very rarely one encounters patients who are extremely arrogant, overly demanding, and insensitive to the fact that doctors also need rest, but to simply discharge the patient without assurance that the person can get help elsewhere would be an act of abandonment. This would be both unethical and illegal. The primary physician, or the physician of record, also has the right to have a colleague follow up on a patient's condition during times when the doctor is on vacation or otherwise unavailable, without fear of being accused of abandonment as long as the patient has been informed. Physicians also have the right to place certain reasonable limits upon the demands of the patient. The ill are frequently egocentric and demanding. Physicians need not go beyond what is necessary for good care. When patients demand that their doctor visit them at home when they are perfectly capable of traveling to the physician's office, their doctor not only has the right to refuse, but should refuse, unless he or she is free of time constraints. Physicians have the right to work only within their chosen specialties, except in emergencies, and the right to refuse to start or continue treatment that they believe is not warranted despite a patient's request for such therapy. To do otherwise would tend to erode the most precious attribute of the physician—integrity.

Other than the above rights, the physician is heaped with extensive obligations and duties. These have been summarized in the codes and oaths designated to guide physicians. The attitudes expressed in these codes have been part of the consciousness of physicians throughout the centuries. Prominent within this attitude is the following dictum by Hippocrates in *Epidemics*: "Make a habit of two things—to help, or at least to do no harm."[9] However, this concept must not be taken out of the total context of medical treatment. Adequate therapy frequently demands temporary discomfort and risk. This was always known, but not always accepted. Each and every medical equation must balance the value of therapy against the potential for undesirable side effects. Each and every ordinary X-ray causes minuscule damage to the body, so small that it cannot be adequately measured. Every brain and heart operation may result in death. Many patients never sense the anguish surgeons may feel worrying about the risk their patients must face. Risk is never absent in the presence of therapy, so the existence of risk should never, in itself, be the basis upon which the decision to treat or not to treat is made.

Physicians should inform and advise persons in their charge about what they believe to be the medically best course of action and, if warranted, should persuade their patients to accept treatment. Time must therefore be devoted to patients so that insecurities are alleviated if at all possible. Physicians are obligated to do all they can to protect the patients' well-being. This requires dedication to maintain an updated understanding of medicine, to exercise caution in therapy, to seek answers (some of which may elude them) by study and by consultation, to help negate the ever-present lingering doubt in the mind of even the most loyal patient as to the validity of any therapy, and therefore to freely offer consultation. Some patients may feel that a request for consultation would be an affront to their doctor. Physicians must appreciate their dilemma and preempt their hesitancy. Fundamentally, physicians are obligated to avoid doing to patients what the doctors would not want done to themselves if the roles were reversed, as well as refraining from actions that patients do not want performed regardless of the physicians' inclinations. This holds true in relation to informed consent, therapy, and confidentiality. Physicians must appreciate that patients' values may be quite different from their own.

There is a dilemma that occasionally occurs within the hospital setting of which the patient, although intimately involved, is usually unaware. A junior physician, who may be a minor participant in the care of a patient, cannot ignore the rights or safety of the patient even though these may have been ignored by the senior physician. If the junior colleague believes either problem may exist and the patient may be harmed, he or she must bring it to the attention of the senior physician. If the senior refuses to explain, or expresses anger instead of gratitude for the opportunity to correct what may be an oversight, the junior doctor or intern should, in view of his or her lesser experience, discuss the problem with other colleagues. If the fears are confirmed, the hospital director must be informed and, if necessary, the patient should be made aware of the difference of opinion. This demands not only dedication but courage to face possible retribution as a result of the senior physician's anger. The ethics of medicine places physician obligation to the patient above any relationship that may exist with an associate physician working on the same case.

PHYSICIAN'S RISKS

This issue has become more prominent with the onslaught of newly discovered deadly viruses.

The duty of the physician is to help those who are ill. In choosing the medical profession the physician must accept this obligation and its occupational hazards, just as the fireman or policeman does; otherwise he or she is entering the profession under false pretenses.

During past decades, when the relationship between doctor and patient was in the nature of a covenant, the trust and belief in the doctor's integrity were answered by a readiness of the physician to go that extra mile and treat regardless of economics, or danger to self. But with erosion of the covenant both patient and doctor have acquired a sense of greater independence. The parental attitude of the physician toward the patient has deteriorated. This unfortunate change has lessened the degree of selflessness traditionally embodied in the image of the physician. But this deterioration did not and does not reduce the physician's obligation and duty to treat even at risk. The only difference is that now the degree of risk is a more prominent variable in the face of the ever-present underlying concept of self-preservation.

The chance of contracting AIDS during a surgical procedure through contaminated blood via needle stick or spray is very small, but still possible. If one appreciates the minimal element of risk to the surgeon, it becomes difficult to concede that the surgeon has an ethical right, especially if extra precautions are used, to avoid operating on a patient who is in need of surgery. The ethical equation balances the harm to the patient if surgery is not performed against the minimal risk of harm to the surgeon. Even without consideration of the surgeon's obligation to fulfill his mission and his obligation as a member of the human race to act beneficently, the harm to the patient would appear to be greater than the degree of risk to the surgeon. But this does not always hold true. Certain circumstances may warrant a refusal to be exposed to even minor risks if that risk could lead to almost certain death. Minor risk that may lead to death is not equivalent to minor risk of temporary illness or even disability.

If the life expectancy of the patient is minimal (an arbitrary figure of six months or less), then to expose self to even the small risk of contracting AIDS could be considered imprudent. When one balances the potential risk of contracting a deadly disease by the surgeon, let alone the operating-room personnel, against the harm to the patient by allowing the "terminal" patient to die a few months sooner, the scale probably tips in favor of the surgeon who is disinclined to accept the risk. I do not believe that to operate under such conditions would be mandated by ethics. To perform surgery under such circumstances may be considered noble or magnanimous, but would be supererogatory from the point of view of ethics. But beside cases in which the risk may lead to almost certain death, the surgeon is morally obligated to perform surgery even when at risk.

CONFIDENTIALITY

The issue of confidentiality is at the heart of the doctor-patient relationship. Medical codes refer to the need for confidentiality as an element of the covenant of trust between physician and patient. The information given to a physician by a patient is given in confidence and is not for publication or disclosure without consent. This principle is fundamentally derived from the right of privacy,[10] the right of a person to keep inviolate his body, his property, and his thoughts. But as with all rights, the right of confidentiality is qualified.

In the burgeoning explosion of data processing, data supplied by the patient and for the patient are deposited in physicians' offices, hospitals, wards, laboratories, and record rooms. Teams of medical and paramedical personnel add to these records. They check and recheck, scan and reread these records. As a result of the massive accumulation of data, computers are now a major depository of records. The attendants in charge of records may show them only to authorized personnel. The concept of privacy as it applies to medical data is less and less a reality, however.

The involvement of third-party coverage has eroded this privacy even more. Upon patient authorization, the person's data may be sent to insurance companies or governmental agencies. Both certainly have a right to proper accountability of the funds dispensed for medical care; this does not mean unqualified access to all data, but enough to validate hospital and medical costs. Unfortunately, from the patient's point of view this data may not only be retrieved, with the approval of an insurance applicant, but distributed to other insurance companies through an insurance medical information bureau.[11]

An important issue regarding confidentiality arises if the confidence includes knowledge of potential harm to others as a result of the patient's illness. It is at this point that physicians must balance autonomy and its byproduct, privacy, against the common good. This problem is obvious in cases of convulsive disorders where one who drives an automobile risks killing a pedestrian if a seizure occurs while behind the wheel. In such cases, confidentiality must be broken. The potential harm to the common good far outweighs the harm to the patient. Privacy must be overruled in favor of reporting the patient's condition to the motor vehicle department. Cases involving a disease that can be readily transmitted to others are situations in which the common good again becomes very weighty and must be balanced against autonomy and privacy. In the state of California over sixty communicable diseases must be reported to the local health department. In spite of the presumption that autonomy carries greater weight, the possible damage to society if faced with a potential epidemic—e.g., smallpox or diphtheria—warrants a breach of confidentiality for the common good. This issue has become especially prominent in the face of Acquired Immunodeficiency Syndrome (AIDS). Should all hospital patients be tested for AIDS much as they once were routinely tested for syphilis? Should spouses be informed? Should the sexual contacts of an AIDS patient be identified and informed? In view of the lethal nature of this disease, the common good warrants a breach of confidentiality. This breach does not mean dissemination of information to the general public, but only to pertinent health officials and to those in danger of exposure. It is unconscionable for a person infected with the AIDS virus to demand that those exposed to infection not be informed. It should be considered mandatory that all patients be tested for the virus upon admission to hospitals and clinics. The danger of exposing nurses, technicians, and physicians to needle injury and the blood of patients warrants mandatory testing. The right to privacy in the face of such a deadly disease becomes insignificant compared to the importance of common good for society and beneficence toward the potential victim. The curious observer may well ask at this point: If all hospital patients are to be tested, should not all health-care providers be tested as well? On the surface such a question may appear to have an easy answer, but there is a great difference between these two groups. Almost all hospitalized patients must have samples of blood withdrawn for tests. The hospital nurses, technicians, laboratory crews, doctors, orderlies, and those who clean up are constantly exposed to this blood. The exposure to blood during surgery is a constant risk. Patients, however, are not exposed to blood from hospital health-care personnel.

Let us return to the problem of confidentiality. Much less common, but equally important, is data obtained from a patient in confidence which suggests the possibility of criminal harm to others. This problem became a prominent legal issue in 1974, in the Tarasoff case.[12]

In 1967, a college student fell in love with Ms. Tatiana Tarasoff, who did not reciprocate the affection. As a result, the student became so emotionally distressed that psychiatric help was sought. During therapy, he revealed his intent to kill Ms. Tarasoff upon her return from vacation. Two other physicians concurred with the therapist that the man was a danger to the welfare of other people[13] and recommended confining the student for several days of intensive psychotherapy. Within a few days after his confinement, the man appeared rational and promised to stay away from Ms. Tarasoff. Soon thereafter, he was discharged. Two months later, when she returned to school, he killed her. Neither the victim nor her family had been warned. Because the family had not been made aware of the danger to their daughter, a suit for wrongful death was filed against the parties involved. The problem of the duty to warn is discussed in more detail by George Annas.[14]

Let us evaluate this issue within the frame of reference of the four basic factors of ethics. Undoubtedly, disclosure of a patient's intentions without securing the person's consent may hamper or disrupt psychiatric therapy. This could constitute harm to the patient. Second, the patient certainly has the right to assume that thoughts expressed to a psychiatrist will be held in confidence. To break this confidence is to abrogate the patient's right to privacy. This again constitutes harm to the patient.

This double harm to the patient must now be balanced against potential harm to others. Does this potential harm negate or override the patient's right of privacy? How can these harms be balanced? How can we weigh a physician's obligation and duty to the patient against the doctor's civic obligation and duty to another member of society under the doctrine of beneficence? Would there be any doubt about what a physician should do if a patient discloses that a bomb will be placed in the local supermarket? The physician must weigh the degrees of danger and arrive at a value judgment as to how much danger to others warrants a breach of patient confidence. Psychiatrists, other physicians, and priests frequently grapple with such dilemmas.

A similar conflict, but eased by the demands of law, presents itself when a physician reports to the appropriate authorities, without the patient's consent, an illness that may harm society: for example, contagious diseases such as diphtheria or smallpox, or infectious diseases such as syphilis or gonorrhea. The factor that determines what the physician should do is the potential of serious physical harm. Potential harm to society must be understood to override the physician's obligation to the patient.

Although there is no general law that establishes a duty to help someone in danger—only Minnesota and Vermont have enacted such Good Samaritan laws—there is a moral imperative to do so, within the limits described in the preceding chapter. We would not hesitate to nullify the threat of harm to some member of society exposed to disease or a careening automobile. Such a threat is certainly not more ominous than a specific death threat made by one person against another. Therefore, the final court decision, which supported the claim of the Tarasoff family, fell within good moral principles in spite of the added burden it may have placed upon psychotherapists, priests, or any other member of society to whom such confidential information has been divulged.

Another example of a problem involving confidentiality was described by Dr. Lawrence Schneiderman.[15] A patient who developed signs of hereditary muscular dystrophy refused to give his physician consent to inform his divorced wife, who had custody of their three children, about the possible genetic problem facing the children. In spite of a threatened lawsuit for breach of confidence, Dr. Schneiderman informed the patient's former wife about the problem and suggested that her children's physician be alerted. This very courageous and ethical stance fulfills the legal directive established in the Tarasoff decision.

This has become an important issue for physicians confronted by an AIDS patient who refuses to divulge his or her illness to a spouse. Under such circumstances the patient should be informed that confidentiality should and will be broken to protect the lives of others under the moral factors of the common good as well as beneficence.

In essence, confidentiality is a qualified right, a right

that may and should be broken when a specific danger to health or life of others is a "strong" likelihood.

THE OWNERSHIP OF MEDICAL RECORDS

The question of proprietorship of a patient's medical records, although intimately tied to the issue of confidentiality, may, for the sake of clarity, be discussed as a separate subject.

Who has a right to medical records: the physician, the patient, the hospital, the laboratory, or a funding agency (if one is involved)? Do they all have equal rights to the records? Are the rights absolute or qualified?

The claim that the owner of the paper on which medical data is written is therefore the "owner of the record"[16] appears to be weak. If this were true, who would own a record if the patient supplied the physician with several sheets of paper upon which were recorded medical data?

Many reasons are given to prevent patients from gaining access to their own medical files. These include:

1. *Patients may not understand the technical terminology and therefore may misinterpret the data and act in a way detrimental to their own health.* This assumes that data cannot be explained in laymen's terms or that patients are not mature enough to appreciate the existence of risks in health care. But if this were true, how valid is a patient's acceptance of treatment based upon "technical information" provided in order to obtain an informed consent to treat? If there is need to make a medical decision in the future, is not the data in those records pertinent to making an informed decision? Is it not the patient's prerogative to determine what data will be considered in any future decisionmaking process?

2. *Information within the records may be considered by the physician to be detrimental to the psychological health of the patient* (for example, poor prognosis for future health and life). The question then arises: Should not patients be given the opportunity to organize their futures in a more realistic manner? In addition, aren't physicians wrongly transferring their own fears of disaster onto their patients?

3. *Information within the records may have been obtained from third parties in confidence.* Do patients have the right to data not obtained directly or indirectly from them but from a third party? Under these circumstances physicians may have an obligation to keep that information confidential. This is again a dilemma physicians must face. There is no simple solution to the problem. Doctors must balance the degree of harm to the patient and to the third party, and may decide to remove that information from the record.

4. *Information within the records may reveal actions or lack of actions that suggest incompetence or errors in the medical management of the case.* This is a major concern of both physicians and hospitals. Meaningless errors are quite common and can be grasped by a litigious or angry patient to file legal action against a physician or hospital. Occasionally two tablets of a laxative may have been ordered and only one given by the nurse; this, in the minds of some patients, may be the reason for all the complexities and complications of their illnesses.

From the patient's point of view, there are several important reasons for obtaining copies of all medical data. These include:

(a) detection of errors in the medical history or medical management;

(b) having somewhat greater control over what information may (or may not) be transmitted to others interested in such data; and

(c) preservation of medical data. It is a common practice for hospitals and laboratories to destroy records after a certain period of time. It is not uncommon to regret the loss of X-rays taken ten or fifteen years earlier, X-rays that may be of value in the study of a new ailment.

There is an element of legitimacy in most reasons both for prohibiting and for granting patients full access to their medical records. However, there is no need, ethically or legally, to disclose fully all data to a patient *who has not requested it*. But when a patient *does request* access to all data and copies of all records, it becomes quite arbitrary to assume that a patient has a right to an X-ray report but not to the films themselves. The protective intentions of the physician, or the fear of disclosing errors, does not in any way outweigh the patient's right to the actual medical record, including X-rays, or at least to copies of these records. It also includes the right to know to whom that data has been revealed or who may have had access to it. The patient's reasons for desiring these records are not pertinent to the legitimacy of the request. Since the hospital, laboratory, or physician(s) involved have an equal right to these records, the only solution is to produce copies for the patient upon demand. The one aspect that falls into a grey area is that of data obtained from other sources. The right of patients to have access to their records is, like all rights, not absolute or without qualification. It is not uncommon for patients to withhold what they consider embarrassing medical data, such as a past history of syphilis. Their spouse, believing it to be of potential medical importance in the management of the present illness, may in confidence reveal the data to the doctor. It may not be in the best interests of either party to reveal that breach of confidence.

It is quite reasonable that those who fund medical care for others—third-party insurers, for example—have a right to patient data to verify that their funds are not being misused. But since physicians and hospitals may not be aware of contractual agreements, they should not release patient records to third parties without the patient's consent.

When patients are denied access to their medical files, their ability to protect their right of privacy is significantly limited. This conflict must be resolved by the courts in favor of the patient. As the Illinois Appellate Court held in 1974, "The fiducial qualities of the patient-physician relationship require disclosure of medical data to a patient or his agent on request."[17]

The patient's right both to access and copies of personal medical records has been upheld in several court decisions. And in 1974, the Privacy Act established that a patient "be allowed access to that medical record, including an opportunity to see and copy it."[18] The following recommendations have been made by Barbara Kaiser. They warrant serious consideration for federal law. They would both insure patients' rights to access their medical records and reduce the ever-increasing invasion of patient privacy. They include:

> (1) an enforceable right in a subject to see and copy his own records in the hands of any custodian; (2) a reasonable opportunity to point out errors and have them either explained or corrected; (3) reasonable notice of the identity of the person or organization to whom the information will be given, of the purpose for which it is to be given, and the circumstances under which the transfer will be made, if the information is to

be placed in the possession of anyone other than the original custodian; (4) a duty of confidentiality toward the patient that will restrict the power of any holder of health records to publish or share them except as prescribed; and (5) a duty on the part of any custodian of health records to notify the subject of the records whenever it receives a subpoena to produce those records, so that the subject may have an opportunity, consistent with usual due process criteria, to contest the subpoena.[19]

There is an area within the doctor-patient relationship that has no legal overtones but is crucial to good medicine and is in need of constant reemphasis. When patients decide to forego further diagnostic studies or active treatment in the face of a terminal condition, they tend to enter into a communication limbo. Such patients reasonably fear abandonment by the physician and possibly by their families. Many people are inclined psychologically to abandon the dying and elderly, for they symbolize what we want to avoid, namely, death and aging. The dying do not understand the barrier of fear that prevents family and friends from an open, candid, and compassionate discussion of dying with the dying. The result can be excruciating loneliness at the edge of life.

The physician's presence during this period is critical even though active medical treatment is not in the picture. The psychological needs of patients become prominent at this state. It is the physician who can serve as the liaison between the dying patient and the family to help clarify feelings as yet unspoken.

The physician's obligation to help the patient does not end with the last pill. It continues until the patient's end. Who else can better listen, smile easier, and express humor with a dying patient? To cease active treatment should not suggest that physicians cease active care. Patients, at all times, and especially under such conditions, need to feel that their physician is with them.

The dying patient is extremely vulnerable psychologically to irrational assumptions and unwarranted guilt, but probably the most devastating feeling to a dying patient, besides the uneasiness of approaching death, is the fear of psychological, if not physical, abandonment. This specific problem is not adequately discussed during the training of physicians. It is not simply a matter of understanding the feelings of patients; it is important during the training period that future doctors come to grips with their own feelings about death, the importance of accepting an inevitable death of a patient, and the possible devastating effect to patients if they feel abandoned.

NOTES

1. Robert Veatch, "Models for Ethical Medicine in a Revolutionary Age," *The Hastings Center Report* 2, no. 3 (June 1972): 7.

2. *Mohr* v. *Williams,* 104 N.W. 12 (Minn 1905).

3. Lynn Peterson, personal communication, 1990.

4. The law demands that certain diseases be reported to the proper governmental authorities. The law may demand that patients undergo medical therapy or at least quarantine if there is significant danger of contamination to society.

5. Norman Cantor, "A Patient's Decision to Decline Life Saving Medical Treatment," *Rutgers Law Review* 26, (1973): 12.

6. *Pratt* v. *Davis,* 118 Ill. App. 161, 166 (1905) Aff'd, 224 Ill. 30, 79 N.B. 562 (1906).

7. *Natanson* v. *Kline,* 186 Kan 393, 350 p. 2d 1093; also 187 Kan, 186, 354, p. 2d 670 (1960).

8. See chapter 1, note 10.

9. Ray Gifford, "Primum Non Nocere," *JAMA: Journal of the American Medical Association* 238, no. 7 (August 5, 1977): 589–90.

10. Refer to the discussion of privacy in Appendix B.

11. Paul S. Entmacher, "Computerized Insurance Records," *Hastings Center Report* 3, no. 5 (November 1973): 8–10.

12. *Tarasoff* v. *Regents of University of California,* 118 Cal Rept 129, 553-69; also Dennis W. Daley, "Tarasoff and the Psychotherapist's Duty to Warn," *San Diego Law Review* 12, no. 4 (July 1975): 932–51.

13. Ibid. *San Diego Law Review,* p. 933.

14. George J. Annas, "Confidentiality and the Duty to Warn," *Hastings Center Report* 6, no. 6 (December 1976): 6–8.

15. Lawrence J. Schneiderman, "Ethical Dilemma: Should I Break Patient Confidentiality?" *Medical Economics for Surgeons* (September 1983): 100–104.

16. George Annas, L. H. Glantz, and B. P. Katz, *The Rights of Doctors, Nurses, and Allied Health Professionals* (Cambridge, Mass.: Ballinger Publishing Co., 1981), p. 157.

17. *Cannell v. Medical and Surgical Clinics,* 21 Ill. App. 383, 3154 N.B. 2d 278, 280 (Ill. App. Ct. 3d District 1974).

18. Annas, et al., *The Rights of Doctors, Nurses and Allied Health Professionals,* p. 159.

19. Barbara L. Kaiser, "Patients' Right of Access to Their Own Medical Records," *Buffalo Law Review* (1974): 317–30.

4

The Right of Self-Determination

The right to refuse medical treatment, even when it may lead to death, is equivalent to the right to seek medical treatment. Both are derived from the right of free choice, and the right to be left alone.[1] Since the right to seek medical treatment is generally assumed, the emphasis here will be on the right to refuse it, and on the cases in which a physician should or should not comply with the wishes of a patient, or the patient's next of kin, to cease, or refrain from beginning, medical treatment.

In the United States, there is no law requiring a competent person who is ill to seek medical care. It is entirely up to the individual to decide whether to do so as long as that decision does not produce significant harm to others (as in the case of a contagious disease requiring those infected to be quarantined). The average person may not be the best judge of what constitutes significant harm to himself (herself) or to others. Nevertheless, the right not to seek treatment holds true even if the illness will result in death. Therefore, the competent adult already has a right to die simply by not seeking life-sustaining medical care.

Although the state has an interest in the preservation of life, its primary interest vis-à-vis the individual is the pres-

71

ervation of free choice, the preservation of the freedom to decide to live. It is quite common for jurists to mention the preservation of life as a fundamental state interest. This perpetuates a misconception, placing the interest in preserving life above that of freedom of choice. Professor Mark Moore of the Harvard University Kennedy School of Government suggests that the state also has an interest in the preservation of an individual life on the basis of the common good factor, specifically to enhance the will of others to live and thus to reduce the tendency to give in to despair.[2] This concept, although theoretically sound, does not seem pragmatically significant in view of the infrequency of suicides among the seriously ill. Dr. Moore is inclined to weight autonomy and a tenuous common good in favor of the latter. This tends to underplay the hierarchical distance between them. Autonomy—freedom of choice—generally carries more weight as an ethical factor than the "common good."

The courts, in balancing the state interest in preservation of life against the patient's right of free choice, have upheld the right of a person to choose to refuse medical therapy.

> In cases that do not involve the protection of the actual or potential life of someone other than the decision maker, the state's indirect and abstract interest in preserving the life of the competent patient generally gives way to the patient's much stronger personal interest in directing the course of his own life.[3]

In confronting decisions regarding another person's death, it is important for physicians to avoid projecting their own fears on those for whom death brings welcome release. It would be an injustice to do otherwise. Doctors must be alert to the possibility of hiding behind the principle of benevolence to avoid facing the reality of death itself, even if that death is someone else's. There is an understandable tendency to allow personal anxieties to interfere with another person's freedom to choose death. As Max Delbruck, the Nobel laureate, put it: "It seems the more rational we become, the less we become capable of facing death. In our culture, death is a bad word, a scandalous word."[4] But death is a natural process. It is understandable that we resist it and do not accept it gracefully, but what we should resent more and accept less is the inability to experience the joy and serenity of life. If a person's life is filled only with anguish, in spite of all our community support, does society have the moral right to insist that such a person continue to live?

We must question whether death need be a horror, or whether it might be a warranted and welcome relief from an unacceptable life. Life is an awesome phenomenon of much beauty, but it may become inhuman if we attempt to deny its inevitable end. The hopelessly ill and a significant number of the aged who consider their lives to be devoid of meaningful existence, frequently view death with equanimity. As Norman Cousins put it: "Death is not the greatest loss in life. The greatest loss is what dies inside us while we live. The invariable tragedy is to live without dignity or sensitivity."[5] Many people would prefer death if their mental abilities were only slightly below normal. Others feel that life must always be continued regardless of its quality. It is not a question of who is wiser or whose judgment is better. It is not a question of what anyone else may believe. Instead, it is a question of that individual's right to reach a personal decision. But respect of that right does not mean that we are to be indifferent and detached. The physician should always be available for advice, which should be given and considered in the final decision.

In regard to a patient's right to make a decision, an interesting situation was described by Dr. J. Englebert Dunphy, a surgeon.[6] He discussed his approach in the case of his eighty-five-year-old friend, who was "dreadfully crippled from arthritis . . . unable to leave his bed for . . . years . . . still mentally bright and still possessed of a good cardio-vascular system." This patient was bleeding from a duodenal ulcer. Surgery was mandatory in order to save his life. As Dr. Dunphy describes it, "His wife had died some years earlier; he lived alone with a devoted nurse; family members were very devoted—they came to see him occasionally—but in my view he was a prisoner of this dreadful crippling disease. . . . There was no question in my mind that . . . we could have successfully controlled the bleeding and he would have lived for some indefinite period. After examining the man, I told him that I didn't think an operation was indicated under the circumstances. And he looked right at me. If I've ever seen gratitude in a patient's eyes he showed it. He didn't say a word, but a flicker of a smile crossed his face. I . . . talked to the family. I said again I felt we didn't have a proper indication for operation. The man died later that night. I ask the question: Was my action unethical? Should I have prolonged his life for another one, two, three, four, or five years?"

To answer that question, I suggest that Dr. Dunphy's paternalistic approach, admirable as it may be, could have achieved the same result by more properly and actively involving his patient in the decision-making process. For Dr. Dunphy to tell the patient that surgery was not warranted, but that life could be prolonged if surgery were performed, would have given the patient the opportunity to decide. Almost certainly the patient would not have challenged the opinion that surgery was not warranted. Although I fully appreciate Dr. Dunphy's good motivation and paternalistic approach, it can be overdone.

When a person chooses to die, the question always arises as to whether that decision is wise and warranted. There is no doubt that when people seriously consider choosing death they must be under some emotional strain. Certainly emotion affects judgment, but this does not mean that the judgment is inappropriate.

It is always possible that one who is forlorn and devoid

of a sense of meaning and worth may be influenced to consider death seriously. If a person expresses a wish to die and we acquiesce by our moral support, we must ask whether our acquiescence is due to our desire to be relieved of a burden. We must be very conscious of this question and intellectually honest with the answer. Because of this possibility, the depressed, debilitated, alone, and lonely person who is detached from family and society and who wishes to die, but is still capable of meaningful existence and of obtaining pleasure, should receive every available support to make that existence as meaningful as possible. To do otherwise would abrogate our social responsibility to that person. Beneficence mandates social support, but if psychological and social support is not of realistic value, then beneficence may realistically take the form of understanding and accepting the decision.

Many believe that a more ready acceptance of a patient's wish to die by refusing treatment would reduce the public's respect for life. This is highly speculative. We need not exchange a greater respect for freedom and individual rights for compassion and tenderness; they are not mutually exclusive. An acceptance of a patient's decision to die does not mean that society need be less caring or less inclined to influence a patient to live. We should try to persuade and cajole patients to live, but we may not dictate what they should do.

One of the problems in determining when the right of self-determination may be abrogated lies in the interpretation of *significant harm*. This is difficult to measure.

POSSIBILITIES OF SIGNIFICANT HARM

What is the harm that may ensue from a patient's voluntary exit from life by refusal of medical treatment?

Harm to Survivors

Regardless of the circumstances, we must assume that when a person dies, grief is present. In the case of a slowly dying patient, grief may be mixed with a sense of relief, but the relief does not negate some element of grief. Can it be considered so intense, so prolonged, and so harmful as to outweigh the principle of freedom? Does the grief of survivors, which is relatively transient under such conditions, count for more than the harm in the form of anguish to the dying patient, let alone to that person's sense of freedom and independence?

If a child is the survivor, two important factors must be considered: (a) the loss of parental love and guidance, with potentially damaging psychological consequences (but this may not be any more harmful or traumatic than divorce, which society certainly permits); and (b) loss of financial support.

Harm to Society

First is the potential burden upon society to care for minor children due to the unnecessary death of the supporting parent. In actuality this would be extremely rare.

Second, there is the view that refusal of treatment would significantly deplete the population. When we consider how few people refuse to be treated, such an argument in the face of our population growth is nonsensical.

Third are those who contend that refusing treatment devalues life. The argument that allowing one person to choose to die will set a pattern so that others in a similar tragic state would accept death more readily is valid, but this does not necessarily mean that life would be devalued; indeed it might cause greater respect for a person's dignity. We must appreciate the value of an individual's freedom of choice and the dignity within that freedom. To remove the right of self-determination is to degrade that dignity and hence the value of life itself. The inherent value of preserving freedom, which is so precious in all social issues, makes such an argument to negate freedom of choice quite insignificant. To enhance our respect for the dignity of life may well enhance our sensitivity to those people living without any sense of dignity: the homeless, the lonely old, and the hungry.

Finally, critics may point out the loss to the state of needed skills that may be important to the common good. This seems like a reasonable concern, but, on balance, the small gain to society would not warrant the negation of a patient's privacy and freedom of choice. Those seriously ill or debilitated patients who wish to die are almost always beyond their productive years or abilities anyway. One could argue that if the individual were an actively working genius—an Einstein perhaps—the loss to society might override the individual's freedom. Certainly under those circumstances every effort should be made to encourage living, but not because of some possible value to society but because the person is well. To diminish such efforts for a person considered to be of lesser "value" would invoke the dangerous concept that each individual's value would have to be weighed and measured. What would be the scale or yardstick? Who would be the judge?

Harm to Hospital Personnel, Nurses, and Physicians

There may also be emotional harm to other patients and to the hospital personnel who may be exposed to the situation. Much has been made of the emotional stress upon nurses who cannot accept the idea of stopping treatment when life could still be prolonged. I have witnessed such reactions, but I do believe its significance to be exaggerated. Norman Cantor places this in its proper perspective when he called this argument against the right to die "far-fetched."[7]

Doctors face potential legal action from the next of kin when decisions are made to cease therapy. The next of kin may accuse the physician of allowing their loved one to die. Doctors are aware of this possibility and rather than open this Pandora's box, they may continue to treat against their better medical judgment, and sometimes without the patient's consent as well. Although it is not common, there is occasional significant unpleasant tension between the family and physician, unlike the relationship between the doctor and patient. This tension must be handled delicately if one is to avoid stress being transferred to the patient.

There may be varying degrees of psychological harm to the physician who does not wish to feel guilty about the death of a patient. I do not believe this to be a significant factor. Physicians must be aware of their role as agents of the patient. If they do not agree with a competent patient's decision to refuse medical treatment, they have the prerogative of transferring the case to someone else, or if death may ensue and young children are involved, seeking court assistance. Probably the only other time physicians should try to obtain a court order to negate a patient's refusal of treatment is if an incompetent patient could be restored to a normal or near-normal life.

Physicians must respect the patient's right of self-determination unless authorized to do otherwise by the courts. To treat a hospitalized patient without consent would, except in emergency circumstances, be contrary to hospital regulations. Physicians may be censured for such actions.

All of these possibilities for harm must be taken into consideration when assessing whether or not one should seek a court order to negate a patient's request to cease therapy.

LEGAL PRECEDENTS SUPPORTING THE RIGHT OF SELF-DETERMINATION

The right of self-determination in health care, as an outgrowth of freedom and the right of privacy, has been generally upheld by the courts. The following cases involve people who chose to refuse treatment when they were competent.

In 1962, Jacob Dilgard, Sr.,[8] a member of the Jehovah's Witness faith, refused to give his surgeon consent to perform a blood transfusion during an anticipated surgical procedure. He was willing to undergo the surgery and to accept the higher risk of death by his refusal of blood transfusions. Since the decision was contrary to good medical advice, and since the surgeon did not simply wish to refuse to operate, which was his prerogative, the court was asked to intervene and to allow the surgeon to operate with the use of blood without the patient's consent. The court ruled to uphold the individual's basic right of free choice. The court did not use free exercise of religion as a basis for its decision, but freedom itself, which is fundamental to and underlies freedom of religion. If the decision were based upon freedom of religion, it would leave open the question of right of free choice for the nonreligious.

In a similar case,[9] the right of decision making was specifically based upon free exercise of religion. Mrs. Brooks was an elderly woman who refused to accept a blood transfusion on the basis of her religious faith. An appeals court upheld her right to do so since her refusal was made when competent and her death did not present any clear and present danger to society

In both of these cases, the potential harm in the form of sadness to survivors was not deemed significant enough to outweigh the individual's right of self-determination.

The right of self-determination and the right of privacy have been strongly supported by the U.S. Supreme Court since at least 1891, when, in the Union Pacific Railway case, it stated:

No right is held more sacred, or is more carefully guarded, by the common law, than the right of every individual to the possession and control of his own person, free from

all restraint or interference by others, unless of clear unquestionable authority of law.[10]

This respect for privacy was also stressed by Justice Ben-
jamin Cardozo. In 1914, he wrote the now-famous words:
"Every human being of adult years and sound mind has
a right to determine what shall be done with his own body."[11]
Over a decade later, in 1928, Supreme Court Justice Louis
Brandeis addressed this same basic issue:

> The makers of our Constitution . . . sought to protect Amer-
> icans in their beliefs, their thoughts, emotions and their
> sensations . . . they conferred . . . the right to be left alone
> . . . the most comprehensive of rights and the right most
> valued by civilized man.[12]

This was further expounded in 1960 by the Supreme Court
of Kansas in the case of *Natanson* v. *Klein*. Justice Alfred
Schroeder expressed it succinctly:

> Anglo-American law starts with a premise of thoroughgoing
> self-determination. It follows that each man is considered
> to be master of his own body and he may, if he be of sound
> mind, expressly prohibit the performance of lifesaving
> surgery or other medical treatment.[13]

As mentioned before, however, this right of free choice
may be negated if significant harm may result. Is the unnecessary death of a parent tantamount to abandonment
of a child? Will the child be emotionally harmed to a significant degree? Will the youngster become a burden upon
society? In other words, do parents have the right to impose
harm upon strangers in society in the form of support for
the children they leave behind? This is obviously a grey area
of decision making that may lead to the negation of an
individual's right to refuse medical treatment.

This problem was discussed in 1972 in the Osborne case.[14] The opinion, written by Judge J. Nebeker of the District of Columbia Court of Appeals, upheld a prior decision. It involved a thirty-four-year-old man who refused a blood transfusion on religious grounds. He preferred to die rather than be given blood which would deprive him of "life everlasting" in heaven, even if he received blood involuntarily.

> Judge Bacon took note of a possible overriding state interest based on the fact that the patient had two young children. It was concluded, however, that the maturity of this lucid patient, his long standing beliefs and those of his family did not justify state intervention . . . a close family relationship existed which went beyond the immediate members, and that the children would be well cared for, and that the family business would continue to supply material needs.

In this grey area, one cannot dogmatically assume that the harm to the children due to the loss of their father (or mother) constitutes a greater or lesser harm to the parent who may continue to live with the belief that he or she can never attain "life everlasting." This balance of harm against harm is independent of balancing the potential harm upon the children against the patient's autonomy. If I had been the judge, I believe I would have insisted upon the use of blood since I believe the loss of a father would constitute greater harm. In this grey area there is no absolute right or wrong.

In a similar situation, Judge Timothy Murphy of the Superior Court of the District of Columbia decided that the problem of child abandonment, even though the child was an infant, was not significant enough to override a mother's refusal to receive blood.[15]

On the other hand, in a more complex situation, blood transfusions were ordered to be given to a twenty-five-year-old mother who was in dire need of blood following an accident. She had a seven-month-old child. Transfusions were refused on religious grounds supported by the right of free choice. The woman's husband agreed with and supported his wife's decision. The court also supported the patient's right to refuse blood. But the decision was overruled and blood was ordered to be given by Circuit Court Judge J. Skelly Wright.[16] He visited the critically ill patient and heard her say that to give blood would be against her will, but when he rephrased the question, "She indicated . . . that (if the court ordered it), it would not then be her responsibility."

This is a situation where the decision to force the use of blood did not need to be made on the basis of harm to a child as a result of unnecessary abandonment. The other factor was benevolence toward the patient. It was quite reasonable to assume that the patient would wish to live if she could be relieved of responsibility for the decision. She might well have appreciated it that Judge Wright ordered blood against her "expressed" desires. Under such a condition, court interference to preserve the life of a young mother would appear reasonable. It would indeed be tragic for a person ambivalent about death to die because of a religious encumbrance when intervention by another person could solve the problem. Therefore, to err on the side of safety and to invoke the doctrine of benevolence to preserve life was reasonable.

This psychological ambivalence did not exist in the decision-making process of Judge Murphy. He stated that, "There was not a scintilla of evidence that she wavered in any way from a decision not to receive blood."[17] In such cases, if the surviving parent or relatives could not, or would not, be willing to assume care of the child, the argument can be made that the child could be harmed as a result of the loss of its mother and that the child could become a burden upon society The refusal of treatment could result in an unacceptable imposition upon society and be considered productive of unwarranted harm to the community. The patient does not have the right to transfer to society, without society's consent, her responsibility toward her child.

In the preceding paragraphs, we explored the principles involving the adult who made a decision while competent and who remained competent. Let us discuss a second category, an adult who made a decision while competent, but who subsequently became incompetent. Should the decision be honored if it can be considered foolish and likely to cause death?

In 1973, Mrs. M. Yetter refused surgery to remove a cancer of the breast despite a good chance for a cure. She understood that her refusal would almost certainly lead to death. As the months went by, she became delusional and was eventually considered incompetent. Her brother requested court authorization to have the surgery performed now that she was incompetent. The court denied the request on the basis that "the constitutional right of privacy includes the right of a mature competent adult to refuse to accept medical recommendations that may prolong one's life," and that, in spite of the risk of death, in order to ensure "the greatest possible protection to an individual in furtherance of his own desires we are unwilling now to overrule Mrs. Yetter's original . . . competent decision."[18]

In 1972, a Jehovah's Witness patient in need of blood refused to receive a transfusion.[19] Her husband and son supported her decision. Within one week she became comatose, at which time she was obviously incompetent. At that time a request was made to the court to negate her decision and to permit the blood transfusion.

Judge Sullivan, after full deliberation, denied the husband's request. Although he personally disagreed with the patient's wish, the judge could not impose "his personal opinions upon an adult competent citizen." The patient subsequently died.

The preceding two cases reflect the wishes of the court

to hold individual freedom most precious. Under these circumstances, the single most crucial issue is to determine if the patient, when competent, expressed a decision regarding the use or nonuse of medical therapy. If such a decision has been expressed in writing as a "directive" to the physician, it must be honored, as was Mrs. Yetter's in the preceding case. If the physician wishes to challenge the directive, then legal support must be sought. That was precisely why I introduced the concept of a "Directive to the Physician" in 1975. A directive is not simply a request. It is an order. If the physician ignores it, he or she is in jeopardy of legal action. Only the court has the legal right to counteract a patient's written directive.

If physicians are aware of such a directive prior to the condition of incompetency and continue to accept and care for the patient, then they are morally obligated to treat or not to treat as directed by the patient. If a court order is sought to negate the "directive" after the patient becomes incompetent, then the physician in question must admit to having accepted the case under false pretenses in the first place. However, if the doctor is unaware of such a previous directive and is suddenly presented with it after the patient has become incompetent, and if the doctor disagrees with the decision, there is a professional obligation to seek court assistance to negate the directive. Legally as well as morally the physician is bound not to treat unless granted the right to do so by the court.

If the courts were to negate a competent person's wishes after the individual becomes incompetent, what would this imply regarding the validity of wills? Competency is certainly lost with death.

A third category of cases pertains to mental incompetents who have never been in a position to state what their desires would be or who have never, even by innuendo, suggested what those wishes would be. Who is to act as a surrogate voice? How is this to be done? Who is in the best position to make a decision for an incompetent individual? A judgment must be made, for to continue the status quo is to make a judgment by default.

If physicians respect the dignity of incompetents, they must appreciate the uncertainty surrounding decisions to treat or not to treat, since these decisions may or may not be in accord with the dignity that medical professionals purport to respect. This places some members of society in an uncomfortable decision-making position.

At present, a conflict exists as to how one may reach a decision affecting an incompetent person. The debate, both legal and philosophical, revolves around two separate legal concepts: "substituted judgment" and "best interests." Since these are not clearly defined concepts, there are variations to both.

The "substituted judgment" doctrine directs itself toward determining what decision an incompetent patient *would* make if he or she were competent and aware of all data pertinent to the present medical situation. The pertinent ethical factor is autonomy since each person, competent or incompetent, has a right to choose his or her course of medical treatment.

The "best interests" test, as it applies to bioethics, and as Robert Weir expresses it,

> hangs on the question of whether the medical procedure will on balance harm or benefit the incompetent person. Not on whether the incompetent person would have chosen the procedure had he or she been capable of doing so.[20]

The intended ethical factor is beneficence. In practice the "best interests" standard has been primarily applied to decisions involving infants.

Both doctrines have been used repeatedly in case law with conflicting viewpoints. Richard O'Neal referred to this conflict when he stated that "the courts have often misused" the concepts of substituted judgment and best interests.[21]

But then again, who is to say what is proper or improper use of doctrines that are imprecisely defined? The legal opinions and evaluations have been discussed in depth by Weir,[22] Ramsey,[23] Annas,[24] Macklin,[25] O'Neil,[26] and Robertson.[27]

Let us put aside judicial opinions for the moment and discuss the problems raised by the substituted judgment concept. Many ethicists and physicians believe that the reasonable substituted-judgment test should be reserved for those patients who have in some way indicated what their wishes would have been under their present set of circumstances. The test is directed toward confirming this wish. It is based on the understanding that the incompetent person has the same right of decision making as the competent person and that autonomy is a primary ethical factor equalled in importance only by the factor of nonmaleficence. As stated by Massachusetts Supreme Court Justice J. Liacos:

> The principles of equality and respect for all individuals
> . . . must extend to the case of an incompetent, as well as
> a competent patient because the value of human dignity
> extends to both. . . .
>   To presume that the incompetent person must always
> be subjected to what many rational and intelligent persons
> may decline is to downgrade the status of the incompetent
> person by placing a lesser value on his intrinsic human
> worth and vitality.[28]

There should be no significant conflict in the use of the substituted judgment doctrine if patients, when competent, have expressed in some way what their desires would be if ever they became incompetent. But even this can be twisted to satisfy preconceived ideas, or political pressures. The *Cruzan* decision,[29] which demanded an unreasonable degree of "clear and convincing" evidence of a patient's wishes, reflected the psychological slant of the U.S. Supreme Court justices to treat someone in a persistent vegetative state in spite of her parent's unchallenged statement that to continue treatment would be contrary to the patient's wishes. It is precisely in the management of such patients whose prior attitude toward medical care when in their present state is not in writing or incontestable, that serious problems arise regarding the use of the "substituted judgment" standard.

Bioethicist Ruth Macklin places stringent limitations upon proxy decision making. She states that for substituted judgment to be valid the representative for an incompetent person must have "individualized, subjective knowledge of the incompetent."[30] This position is supported by O'Neil, Weir, and Paul Ramsey. Ramsey follows this position with a statement that, unless their desires had been previously made known, "incompetent patients do not have 'privacy' in the sense of autonomy or self-determination."[31]

These ethicists therefore prefer to use the "best interests" standard instead of "substituted judgment" in cases where prior knowledge of a patient's desires are unknown. O'Neil attempts to summarize and validate this approach by suggesting that,

> Respect for autonomy only makes sense when we do have knowledge of actual choices or preferences, we must determine our conduct in these cases by the principle of beneficence and seek the incompetent's best interests.

But then he concedes the danger in its use: "The patient's best interest is subject to various interpretations, including the proxy's own idiosyncratic notion of what would be good for the patient."[32]

Weir's strong condemnation of the use of substituted judgment when there is no prior knowledge of a patient's wishes is explained as follows:

If the substituted judgment test is applied to cases in the
NICU (Neonatal Intensive Care Unit), it takes the form
of asking, "What would infant A choose if infant A could
choose?" Given that an infant has no history of choices,
or even desires or preferences, this attempt at determining
the validity of proxy consent or denial of consent for infants
is seriously limited if not impossible. . . . Such an approach
is fatally flawed for the simple reason that no one—especially normal, healthy adults—can place themselves in a
defective newborn's position and view life from that perspective. . . . A much better approach . . . is to use the best
interest test. This test, when applied to the moral decisions
made in the NICU, involves asking, "Would an indefinite
prolongation of life through medical treatment be in the
best interests of infant B?" This second method, specifically
geared to determining whether available treatment would
on balance, be beneficial or harmful to the anomalous neonate, requires utmost care in the diagnosis and prognosis
of the infant's condition, informed judgments regarding
treatment possibilities, and consultation with other persons
in order to arrive at a consensus decision.[33]

But he then concedes that this approach is

open to vacuous concepts of what constitutes best interests and to a proxy's own idiosyncratic notions of what
would be beneficial or harmful for the infant . . . the
possibility of error is unavoidable, but the same is true for
many of the judgments made in clinical medicine.[34]

Weir then proceeds to state that,

Selection by categories of congenital defect affirms the basic
equality of neonates. When decisions are made to withhold
treatment in this manner, it is because a particular neonate
has a medical condition for which there is no beneficial
treatment, not because the infant is judged to be of little
value or to have a life not worth living.[35]

On this basis a lesion or defect that can be treated should be treated regardless of any other defects that may be present. Therefore a severely brain-damaged, paralyzed newborn who would not have bladder or bowel control, and who has an imperforate anus, should have anal surgery in order to prolong life. In whose "best interests" would such an action be?

Because a "best interests" doctrine bypasses the factor of autonomy and attempts to use the factor of beneficence in order to reach a decision, John Arras believes that "the best-interests standard presents staggering problems of interpretation and application,"[36] and since there is a tendency to disregard all variables except the isolated organic medical problem, Arras offers the following suggestion:

> The best-interest standard consigns itself in extreme cases to operating in a moral vacuum. The result is an indiscriminate mandate to treat, to keep alive, that flies in the face of common sense.[37]

This pitfall, so evident in Weir's approach, is reflected in a statement by Ramsey: "Medical criteria for care should remain physiological. . . . Decision to treat or not to treat should be the same for the normal and the abnormal alike."[38] Therefore, quality of life is never to be considered.

To design this type of a decision-making process, which considers only one medical factor and ignores others as well as ignoring social factors, suggests a psychological need to avoid the unpleasant decision to allow life to end. In real life, rational, competent people do not make decisions on only one factor when several factors may apply, even though the decision-making process may be difficult. Richard McCormack makes the following observation: "As social beings, our good, our flourishing (therefore our best interests) is inextricably bound up with the well-being of others."[39] It would be absurd to assume that a specific physical gain to myself at the expense of devastating social effects upon my children could be construed as in my best interests. According to McCormack, "Something can be, therefore, in our best interests without we ourselves, precisely as isolated individuals, deriving any benefits or gains."[40]

The fact that a patient may be in a state during which the exercise of free choice cannot be accomplished does not negate the person's right to expect society to carry out that choice on his or her behalf. To hide behind the assumption that we cannot transpose ourselves into the incompetent patient's mind makes the unwarranted assumption that the patient, if competent, would approve that a vital decision be made without regard to all relevant factors simply because to do so would be difficult or onerous. This would be a most unreasonable assumption. By ignoring certain factors, we take the liberty of utilizing only those factors which satisfy our personal beliefs. This approach does not portray beneficence but rather an unconscious fear of responsibility or an unwarranted self-righteousness to support a preconceived decision based upon a psychological view that life must always be preserved. If the "best interests" standard ignores important parameters, such as the quality of life, then physicians would be treating an incompetent person in a manner wholly unlike the way they would treat someone who is competent. This would be placing a lesser value on the intrinsic worth of an incompetent person. There is a heavy burden of proof upon the shoulders of those who insist on using such an approach.

If substituted judgment is only to be used when there is already knowledge of what the patient desires, the judgment is not truly substituted judgment, but rather a substantiation, in reality only a surrogate confirmation of a prior decision. Reasonable substituted judgment only has true significance when we are unaware of what the patient's decision would have been. When we view an incompetent individual as an intelligent, competent adult we portray respect of that individual's autonomy and thereby act in that individual's best interests. It is, according to Robertson, "in the incompetent's best interest to be treated as nearly as possible as the person he would be."[41] To act accordingly is, if anything, to err on the side of safety. It would be dangerous to allow others to superimpose their ideas of what is best above what would reasonably have been made if the patient had been competent and aware of all data.

It is more reasonable to assume that any person, regardless of age—and that includes the conceptus on into old age—would want society to make a substituted decision that would assume (1) they have been or would eventually become at least of average intelligence, and (2) they would be rational adults who would take all factors into consideration prior to reaching a decision. We should appreciate that the conceptus-fetus-newborn is directed toward becoming a rational adult and would want to be respected as a potential adult. Obviously when decisions are made that may have social impact, patient priority is paramount regardless of the patient's age. However, establishing priorities does not deny the need to consider all factors.

This broad view of the substituted-judgment approach, one that considers all variables, is the clearest way to achieve the best-interest result regardless of the age of the patient. Medical decisions demand consideration of all variables. If we do otherwise, we enter a pitfall where personal bias may decide what variable to select. Massachusetts Justice Liacos supports this position since " 'best interests' devalues that person's humanity by ignoring the subjective wishes and circumstances of the individual on whose behalf the decision is ostensibly being made."[42]

The Saikewicz case illustrates the issues that arise in such a situation; the principles here apply to all incompetent people whose desires are unknown.[43]

In 1976, Joseph Saikewicz, a sixty-seven-year-old severely retarded resident of a state institution, was diagnosed as having acute myelomonocytic leukemia.* His mental age was below three, and his mental status was irreversible. If the illness is left untreated, the average survival period is approximately four months. The chemotherapy for this condition has unpleasant side effects. It necessitates three to six weeks in the hospital for intensive chemotherapy, which offers approximately a 50 percent chance to prolong life for one year. The state facility had an important question to address: Should the patient receive chemotherapy to prolong life? There were no family members to assist in the decision.

The superintendent of the state school asked the courts to appoint a guardian to make the decision whether to treat or not to treat. One might ask why such a request was necessary. George Annas expresses the reason quite well:

> Judges are asked to decide . . . (whether or not life-sustaining treatment should or should not be withheld from patients who are unable to make the decisions themselves) not because they have a special expertise but because only they can provide the physicians with civil and criminal immunity for their actions. In seeking this immunity, legal considerations quickly transcend ethical and medical judgments.[44]

Before proceeding to the legal ramifications, let us make the assumption that most competent people who have such a disease would probably wish to be treated in spite of some of the undesirable side effects of chemotherapy and the relatively short period that life may be prolonged. Second, we may assert that if Mr. Saikewicz were competent he would have the prerogative of accepting or rejecting the treatment program.

If we apply our four moral factors to this case, it is

---

*An incurable disease of the white blood cells. Life can be prolonged with treatment.

apparent that whether or not Mr. Saikewicz were able to decide for or against chemotherapy, no significant harm to others would be caused. Certainly, prolonging his life by treating him would be an expense for society and therefore an imposition and possible harm. However, this expense is quite insignificant when weighed against a concern for life.* Therefore, the factors of harm to others and the common good are essentially not relevant. The factor of beneficence is relevant only in the sense that we must act in the patient's best interests and try to decide what the patient would wish if he were able to express his desires.

Since we cannot be certain, we must consider what most people would view as reasonable and would wish to have done or not done to themselves under similar circumstances. What directive would most people write to their physician, when competent, if aware that they were to become permanently incompetent with a mental age of three and suffer from leukemia? Would they direct the doctors to prolong their life at that point or to refrain from prolonging it? Do we have any reason to assume that Mr. Saikewicz would not wish, if he were able, to fall into the category of "most" people? If so, then we must reevaluate the question and tailor it specifically for the person in question. If there are no reasons to assume that special factors would exist, then what would be sufficient and reasonable to most people must be considered applicable to Mr. Saikewicz. In the opinion of Massachusetts Justice Liacos, the "substituted judgment" principle "commends itself simply because of its straightforward respect for the integrity and autonomy of the individual."[45] In essence, as expressed by Justice Liacos,

> We realize that an inquiry into what a majority of people would do in circumstances that truly are similar assumes an objective viewpoint not far removed from a "reason-

---

*This will be discussed in more detail in chapter 10, on triage.

able person" inquiry . . . we should make it plain that the primary test is subjective in nature—that is, the goal is to determine with as much accuracy as possible the wants and needs of the individual involved. This may or may not conform to what is thought wise or prudent by most people.[46]

Who has, or should have, the right to use reasonable "substituted judgment" when dealing with incompetent patients? The Supreme Court of New Jersey suggests that the

practice of applying to a court to confirm such a decision would generally be inappropriate not only because it would be a gratuitous encroachment upon the medical profession's field of competence, but because it would be impossibly cumbersome.[47]

Unless there are highly extenuating circumstances, "substituted judgment" decisions regarding medical treatment should remain within the domain of the medical profession and the patient's guardian or family. The immediate next of kin—spouse, offspring, and, to a lesser degree, parents and siblings—are closer in relationship and should be more responsible for decision making than the physician. Their authority, although not absolute, is to be respected more than the authority of the physician unless there are extenuating circumstances. The courts have confirmed the right of immediate family members to act as surrogates for the patient, including the right to order cancellation of medical treatment on behalf of the patient within the constraint that the motivation must be one of concern for the patient. Next-of-kin decisions can be made without prior judicial approval.[48] If the next of kin believe, as a result of their knowledge of the patient, that the patient would want treatment to stop, then, in their capacity to act for the patient, they are obligated to demand that treatment be stopped. The physician must then reflect upon whether the patient's desires would be the same. Does the attitude of next of kin truly reflect the attitude of the patient? If so, the physician must not continue therapy, not because of the next of kin's demand, but because he or she accepts their statement that they honestly believe this is what the patient would want and that the request is medically reasonable. But if the physician believes, in his or her "substituted judgment" for the patient, that the patient would not wish therapy to be stopped, then the doctor is ethically bound, within the framework of the covenant and as the agent of the patient, to seek a court order granting the right to treat. Such court approval is necessary to protect the patient from overzealous physicians and to protect doctors from litigious next of kin.

There is an important aspect in this line of reasoning that needs further discussion. The emphasis should not be on the *result of a decision* but rather *the right in a free society to make a decision*. It is not a question of whether we have a right to live or a right to die. Instead, it is a question of whether we have the right to *decide* to live or to *decide* to die. It is the right to make a free choice that is crucial. Benjamin Friedman speaks precisely to this crucial point. He states that, "The value of a right to freedom does not lie in the content given to the right but in the act of exercising the right.[49]

We must be aware of certain dangers inherent within "substituted judgments," whether exercised by the family, the physician, or the courts. It is obvious that misuse of "substituted judgment" can be deadly. Many institutionalized incompetent people could be denied treatment without good reason. One criterion should be mandatory in such decision dilemmas. If the incompetent person is conscious enough to express, by action or by word, a desire to be treated, *treatment must be given, even if competent, reasonable, "substituted judgment" would deem treatment to be unwarranted.*

WRITTEN DIRECTIVES TO PHYSICIANS

We have explored some of the problems, both moral and legal, that arise in attempting to respect a person's right of self-determination. How can some of these problems be avoided? How can patients express their wishes and establish a more precise understanding with their physicians? How can we protect the patient's wishes and, at the same time, allay the physician's fear of criticism or prosecution when complying with those wishes?

This problem must be discussed with candor. Much of the time, when physicians oppose patients' requests or the requests of next of kin, their opposition is based more on fear of legal reprisal than on moral drive. Pseudoethical considerations are frequently used as an excuse to hide the fear that legal action might be instituted by some member of the patient's family or by the local district attorney on the fallacious assumption that physicians are always obligated to treat.

It must be reemphasized that the physician is the agent and benefactor of the patient and is obligated to help while still respecting the patient's desires. This does not necessarily mean that the doctor should set about a course of treatment.

This obligation is less difficult to fulfill if patients expressly state their desires, preferably in written form, when competent. If patients are not physically able to write their wishes but are still mentally competent, their desires can be written for them in the presence of witnesses. It is important to realize that patients have the right of decision making with or without a specified directive and with or without legislative acts to support such directives. The following is an example of such a document:

DIRECTIVE TO MY PHYSICIAN

This declaration applies to all involved in my care, especially my family, my physicians or any physician in charge of my care, my attorneys, and the medical facilities involved.

This directive is written while I am of sound mind and fully competent.

If, at any time, I become incompetent, regardless of the cause, in consideration of my constitutional and legal right to refuse medical or surgical treatment regardless of the consequences to my health and life, I hereby direct and order my physician or any physician in charge of my care, to cease and refrain from any medical or surgical treatment that would prolong my life if I am in a condition of:

1. unconsciousness from which I cannot recover, or in a persistent vegetative state; or

2. mental incompetence which is irreversible. (However, if, although I become mentally incompetent, I am still able to converse and to partially understand, I must be openly informed of the situation and, if I wish to be treated in my incompetent state, I am to be treated in spite of my original request made while competent.)

Under the above circumstances, the only treatment to be given may be sedation and analgesics for relief of distress. Any form of artificial ingestion of food or water is forbidden.

If there is any reasonable doubt of the diagnosis and prognosis of my illness, then consultation with available specialists must be obtained. If any action is taken contrary to these expressed demands, I hereby request my next of kin or my legal representative to take legal action against those involved for assault and battery and malpractice for treating me without my consent.

I hereby, for myself, my heirs, executors, administrators and personal representatives, absolve and relieve my physician or any physician taking care of me, or any hospital or

sanitarium or extended care facility at which I may be at
the time of my illness, from any legal responsibility pertaining to the fulfillment of any of my demands.

_____
Signature

_____
Date

Witness _____

Witness _____

There are two reasons for such a strongly worded directive:
first, to unequivocally express how the patient wishes to be
treated, and second, to protect the physician. By expressing a specific intent to seek legal action against anyone
who countermands the directive, the physician is placed in
a position of jeopardy. No one can reasonably expect physicians to place themselves in such a position. Therefore, the
treating physicians are both psychologically and legally
supported if they are in agreement with the patient's
demands to stop treatment. If the physicians receive this
directive after incompetence has been reached and if they
believe the demands are unwarranted, then their only
recourse is to seek court approval to treat without the
patient's consent.

To this date no action has been brought against a
physician or medical facility for withholding or cancelling a
medical program at the request of a patient. Recent court
decisions have upheld that documents of this nature may
be relied upon by physicians and health facilities without
further judicial advice.[50]

An alternative approach would be for patients to grant

specified persons unquestionable right to speak for them if ever incompetence is established; to appoint persons to act as their attorney in fact in regard to health care. This would constitute a "durable power of attorney."[51] It is in many ways another form of the directive to physicians. The signer of the document may state which conditions should or should not be treated, or the signer may leave out specific details with the understanding that the surrogate voice fully appreciates the signer's desires.

A well-written, witnessed, and preferably notarized "Directive to Physicians would be equally effective.

A "durable power of attorney" document can be a simple statement such as:

I, ____name____ , appoint ____person of choice____ to act as my attorney-in-fact to make all decisions for me regarding my health care if I become incompetent. This includes the right to order my physician and medical facility to cease all treatment that would maintain life.

Date _____ Witness _____ Witness _____

Signed _____

Once this type of authorization has been given, the next of kin or whoever has been appointed attorney-in-fact can present the physician and/or medical facility with a "limitation of consent to treat" in the event that the patient becomes incompetent. The directive and durable power of attorney may need to be modified according to the laws of the patient's state. The President's Commission for the Study of Ethical Problems in Medicine and Biomedical and Behavioral Research encouraged the use of such documents.[52]

If a directive to the physician or a durable power of attorney has not been executed, then the next of kin may cancel therapy if they are aware of what the patient would wish. In order to expedite such a demand, a letter of authorization would be appropriate. The following suggested letter of authorization may be used.

NEXT OF KIN AUTHORIZATION
AND LIMITATION OF CONSENT TO TREAT[54]

Date _____

I (We), the wife, husband, son, daughter, brother, sister, father, mother, grandfather, grandmother, guardian, being fully competent, authorize all doctors, nurses, technicians or other personnel involved in the treatment of our _____relationship_____ to cease all treatment except medication for sedation and control of discomfort. We insist that you allow nature to take its course.

I (We) fully understand that beyond any medical probability, there is no reasonable expectation of recovery from the state of severe mental incompetency, or unconsciousness. This letter of authorization limiting the medical and surgical management is not simply our wish but is the expressed wish and demand of_____name of patient_____, who has informed us of his/her wishes and demands, when fully competent.

If this authorization and limitation of treatment as expressed by _____name of patient_____ through us is not respected, we shall seek legal redress for assault and battery and malpractice for treating without the consent of the patient.

_____
Signature

_____
Signature

Witness _____

Witness _____

If the physician has reason to doubt the honesty and intent of the next of kin, then professional ethics require seeking court approval to manage the case as the physician believes would be best for the patient.

It is hoped that the public will view directives for medical care as they do wills pertaining to disposition of their estates, and will write, while healthy, a directive to their physician. This would obviate the unpleasant involvement of next of kin in court proceedings.

In essence, if such documents are written and respected, the patient or the patient's family will not be placed in the position of seeking an injunction to stop hospital personnel or physicians from starting or continuing a treatment program. The physician and the hospital administration must never have, except in emergency situations, the right to start or continue treatment without the patient' s direct or "substituted" consent unless granted that right by a court directive.

A BREAKING OF THE RULE

During a discussion of bioethics I had been asked what I would do if a young man of twenty had been brought to an emergency room for a problem that demanded surgical interference for survival. The surgery itself carried only a small risk. The patient was completely conscious, wide awake, had no apparent apprehension or fright, and was intelligent and socially responsive. After discussion of the problem the patient adamantly refused surgery, although he understood that the chances of survival without surgery were extremely small. His reasons for refusal were based primarily upon fear of surgery resulting from an unsuccessful surgical experience within his family.

In this situation I would use any modality, even sedation if necessary, to move ahead with surgery without consent if I could avoid legal implications for the hospital, or, if necessary, without alerting the hospital of the dilemma. How can I say this in view of my respect for individual autonomy? What is my frame of reference?

Rules and regulations, moral principles, axioms, and laws are crucial for a harmonious society. But what is ethically and legally correct as a sweeping generalization may not always be specifically applicable to each individual case. In this particular situation, although the patient was obviously legally competent, I would not consider his "decision-making capacity," to use Wanzer's[54] phrase, as adequate. The consequence of his unreasonable fear would be too tragic. Consequently, I would be making a judgment about competence in the spirit of the law although not within the technical requirements of the law.

As a physician I still feel the presence of a covenant rather than a contract with a patient. I realize this paternalism can be dangerous, but this is exactly what my decision would be if that young man were my son. In balancing the two pertinent factors in this situation, autonomy and beneficence, my antipathy to unnecessary death for someone below the age of thirty would drive me to place beneficence above autonomy and do what is technically illegal. Of course, those who act in a manner outside the law must fully acknowledge the possible penalties associated with their actions.

In spite of divergent legal opinions, as legal decisions have increased, a pattern of legal consensus has emerged. This consensus is summed up by Christopher Armstrong[55] as follows:

> (1) A competent adult has a legal right to refuse medical treatment, a right that may be qualified in particular cases by one of four countervailing state interests.
>
>> (a) The preservation of life.
>>
>> (b) The protection of the interests of innocent third parties.

(c) The prevention of suicide.

(d) Maintaining the ethical integrity of the medical profession.

(2) An incompetent patient has the same right as a competent patient to avoid treatment, and the right may be exercised on his behalf by an appropriate surrogate.

(3) The family of an incompetent patient is presumptively an appropriate surrogate to act on his behalf.

(4) Court proceedings are generally unnecessary to secure approval of a decision to withhold or withdraw life-sustaining medical treatment, except in cases of dispute or where the incompetent patient lacks an appropriate surrogate to act in his behalf.

(5) The entry of a no-code (or DNR—do not resuscitate) order on a patient's chart does not require prior judicial approval.

(6) A decision to terminate medical treatment is subject to the same legal standards as a decision not to begin the treatment.

(7) Rules concerning withdrawal of treatment apply equally to withdrawal of nutrition and hydration by artificial means.

(8) A physician or hospital acting in good faith will not be held civilly or criminally liable for acquiescing in the wish of the patient's family that artificial life-support measures be terminated.

NOTES

1. See Appendix B for a discussion of privacy.
2. Professor Mark Moore, personal communication, 1990.
3. *In Re Conroy,* 464, A. 2d 303, rec'd 486 A. 2d.1209, p. 1223 (N.J. 1985). There is an excellent discussion of state's interest by Norman Cantor in "A Patient's Decision to Decline Life-saving Medical Treat-

ment: Bodily Integrity Versus the Preservation of Life," *Rutgers Law Review* 26 (1973): 238–64.

4. Max Delbruck, "Education for Suicide," *Prism* (November 1974):18.

5. Norman Cousins, *Saturday Review* (June 14, 1974): 4.

6. J. Englebert Dunphy, "Ethics in Surgery: Going Beyond Good Science," *Bulletin American College of Surgeons* (June 1978): 10.

7. Norman Cantor, "A Patient's Decision to Decline Life-saving Medical Treatment."

8. *Erickson* v. *Dilgard,* 252, N.Y.S., 2d 705,706 (Sup. Ct. 1962) Nassau County.

9. *Estate* v. *Brooks,* 205 N.B. 2d 435 (1965), 32 122 2d 361. See Robert Bryn, "Compulsory Life Saving Treatment for the Competent Adult," *Fordham Law Review* 44 (1975): 1–36.

10. *Union Pacific Railway* v. *Botsford,* 141 U.S. 250, 251 (1891).

11. *Schloendorff* v. *Society of New York Hospital,* 211 N.Y., 125, 127, 129, 105 N.E. 92, 93 (1914).

12. *Olmstead* v. *United States,* 277 U.S. 438, 478, 48 Superior Court 564, 572, 72 L. Ed. 944 (1928).

13. *Natanson* v. *Klein,* 186 Kan. 393, 350 P 2d 1093 (1960).

14. *In Re Charles P. Osborne* 294 S. 2d 372 (1972), p. 374.

15. Judge Timothy Murphy, Sup. Court of Dist. of Columbia, Family Division, November 11, 1974: unpublished notes "In the Matter of Janet Pogue and Infant Pogue."

16. Application of the President and Directors of Georgetown College 331 F. 2d (D.C. Cir.) 377 U.S. 978 (1964), p. 1012.

17. Judge Murphy, unpublished notes "In the Matter of Janet Pogue and Infant Pogue."

18. Dockett #1973-553 Pennsylvania Court of Common Pleas, Northhampton County Orphans Court, 1973.

19. *Re: Phelps* #459-207 (Milwaukee County Ct. filed July 11, 1972).

20. Robert E. Weir, *Selective Nontreatment of Handicapped Newborns* (New York: Oxford University Press, 1984), pp. 197–98.

21. Richard O'Neal, "Determining Proxy Consent," *Journal of Medicine and Philosophy* (November 1983): 389–403.

22. Weir, *Selective Non-Treatment of Handicapped Newborns.*

23. Paul Ramsey, "The Saikewicz Precedent: What's Good for an Incompetent Patient?" *Hastings Center Report* 8, no. 6 (December 1978): 36–42.

24. George J. Annas, "Reconciling Quinlan and Saikewicz: Decision

Making for the Terminally Ill Incompetent," *American Journal of Law and Medicine* 4, no. 4 (1979): 367–96.

25. Ruth Macklin, "Return to the Best Interests of the One Who Speaks for the Child," in Wm. Gaylin and R. Macklin, eds., *Who Speaks for the Child?* (New York: Plenum Press, 1982), p. 209.

26. O'Neal, "Determining Proxy Consent."

27. John A. Robertson, "Organ Donations by Incompetents and the Substituted Judgment Doctrine," *Columbia Law Review* 76 (1976): 48–78.

28. *Superintendent of Belchertown State School* v. *Joseph Saikewicz Mass.*, 370 N.B. 2d 417, pp. 427, 428.

29. *Cruzan* v. *Director, Missouri Dept. of Health* 110 S.Ct. 2841 (1990).

30. Macklin, "Return to the Best Interests of the One Who Speaks for the Child," p. 209.

31. Ramsey, "The Saikewicz Precedent: What's Good for an Incompetent Patient?" p. 37.

32. O'Neal, "Determining Proxy Consent," p. 397.

33. Weir, *Selective Non-Treatment of Handicapped Newborns*, pp. 198–99.

34. Ibid., p. 199.

35. Ibid., p. 211.

36. John D. Arras, "Toward an Ethic of Ambiguity," *Hastings Report* 14, no. 2 (April 1984): 26.

37. Ibid., p. 31.

38. Paul Ramsey, *Ethics at the Edges of Life* (New Haven, Conn.: Yale University Press, 1978), p. 206.

39. Richard A. McCormack, "Freedman on the Rights of the Voiceless," *Journal of Medicine and Philosophy* 3, no. 3 (1978): 212–13.

40. Ibid.

41. Robertson, "Organ Donations by Incompetents and the Substituted Judgment Doctrine," p. 58.

42. Paul J. Liacos, "Is Substituted Judgment a Valid Legal Concept?" Lecture for National Legal Center for the Dependent and Disabled, Inc. (April 13,1989), p. 10.

43. *Superintendent of Belchertown State School* v. *Joseph Saikewicz, Mass.*, 370 N.B. 2d 417.

44. George J. Annas, "Judges at the Bedside: The Case of Joseph Saikewicz," *Medicolegal News* 6, no. 1 (Spring 1978): 10–13, p. 10.

45. *Superintendent of Belchertown State School* v. *Joseph Saikewicz*, p. 431.

46. Ibid., p. 430.

47. Annas, "Reconciling Quinlan and Saikowicz," pp. 367–96.

48. *Barber* v. *Superior Court* 2 Civil #69350 2 Civil #69351 Calif. Court of Appeals, Second Appellate District, Division 2, October 1983 (Interim Citation 83 Daily Journal DAR 2841).

49. Benjamin Friedman, "On the Right of the Voiceless," *The Journal of Medicine and Philosophy* 3 (1978): 211–21, p. 207.

50. Matter of *Saunders* v. *State of New York* 129 Misc. 2d 4S New York 1985; *Lurie* v. *Samaritan Health Service Company* Na CS10198 Superior Court, Mariposa Co. Arizona 1984; *John F. Kennedy Memorial Hospital, Inc.* v. *Bludworth* 432 So 2d 611 Reversed 452 So 2d 921 (Fla. 1984).

51. See Appendix C.

52. President's Commission for the Study of Ethical Problems in Medicine and Biomedical and Behavioral Research, *Deciding to Forego Life Sustaining Treatment* (Washington, D.C.: U.S. Government Printing Office, 1983), p. 144.

53. This is a modification of a form proposed by Philip Rossman, M.D., Santa Monica, Calif., in November 1974.

54. S. H. Wanzer et al., "The Physician's Responsibility Toward Hopelessly Ill Patients," *The New England Journal of Medicine* 320, no. 13 (March 30, 1989): 845.

55. Christopher J. Armstrong, "Judicial Involvement in Treatment Decisions," in J. M. Civetta, R. W. Taylor, and R. R. Kirby, eds., *Critical Care* (Philadelphia: J. B. Lippincott Co., 1987), pp. 1649–55.

5

Suicide

The definition of suicide is not clear cut. The ambiguities surrounding the word are due in large part to the negative connotation that contemporary society has given it. Although suicide is generally considered to be an act of intentionally killing oneself, broadly speaking, suicide may be considered to occur when an individual deliberately and knowingly acts in a manner that produces his or her own death regardless of primary motivation or methodology. The father who sacrifices his life in order to save his child does not wish to commit suicide. When the primary motivation is to die, the act in all cases is tied to duress. One does not commit suicide simply to end life, but to end the pains or indignities of life.

Under a broad definition suicide may be accomplished by interfering with natural biological processes, e.g., by an overdose of sleeping pills, or by allowing the natural biologic process to continue to death, by refusal of medical therapy. Suicide can be active or passive, an act of commission or an act of omission. The motivation may be self-serving—a spiteful act to harm the survivor(s)—or an act of altruism, as when a soldier throws himself on a grenade to protect his comrades. Then again, suicide may be to protest social ills, to avoid insulting God, to avoid degradation, or to avoid physical or mental anguish. It may be the result of free choice or limited choice. To die by suicide when sentenced to death by hanging is an extremely limited choice.

Except possibly for those whose religious views lead them to believe that death brings them to greater glory, suicide always occurs during periods of duress. The only common denominators in this broad view of suicide are that death is allowed to occur and that there is some duress. Even the most rational suicide contains an element of distress.

Suicide may be defined as the nonaccidental permitting of one's own life to end, regardless of circumstances or the method used. However, through general usage we are inclined to think of suicide as an active process that immediately or almost immediately results in death. In short, the taking of one's own life. This traditional concept is supported linguistically. The word is derived from the Latin *sui,* or "self," and *cide,* or "killer." *Cide* is derived from *caedere,* which means to kill. *Caedere,* in turn, originates from *skhai,* which means to cut or to strike.[1] This implies an active and immediate effect.

We should, for the sake of clarity, separate the word "suicide" from the word "euthanasia," which is an act whereby one kills another for the benefit of the one who dies. The latter is mercy killing, which will be discussed in chapter 8.

THE BASIS OF THE WESTERN ATTITUDE TOWARD SUICIDE

The most prominent factors that determine our present Western attitude toward suicide are our religious heritage, primarily the Judeo-Christian influence, and peoples' fear of death. Judaism generally condemns suicide. This stems from the first rule in Judaic criminal law expressed in Genesis: "Whoever sheds the blood of man by man shall his blood be shed. . . . For your life blood too, I will require a reckoning."[2]

It is reasonable to assume from the biblical statement that the one who sheds someone else's blood is to be punished by society, while the one who commits suicide will be judged by God. Whether God's punishment will be harsh, lenient, or the act excused is not written.

Certainly the manner of the warning suggests that he who contemplates suicide *may* incur the wrath of God, but the possibility that suicide may be excused by God allowed the Jewish people to assume that under certain extenuating circumstances, God may at least accept the act of suicide. The suicides recorded in both the Old and the New Testaments are mentioned without any suggestion of condemnation toward the persons involved.[3] Suicide is not directly prohibited in either testament.

In spite of the implication that judgment of suicide is only to be made by God, Judaic tradition is inconsistent. It ranges from the prohibition of suicide by Rashi to no prohibition whatsoever by Ibn Izra.[4] Though a general condemnation of suicide existed, Judaism suggests that since every suicide takes place under duress of some form, it may be considered involuntary and therefore excusable. Second, suicide is to be preferred over idolatry, which is considered an insult to God; murder, or killing with malicious intent; as well as incest and adultery. But even these parameters have been broadened.[5] Suicide has been excused as an alternative to torture or expected death, rape, and slavery, and to protect one's people from harm. It has even been excused when committed as a result of extreme devotion to the deceased. There is a story in the Talmud of the laundryman who committed suicide when informed of the death of his beloved rabbi. When this occurred, "A voice resounded from Heaven to invite him to enter Paradise."[6] This suicide was therefore not only excused but lauded. If it was based on severe temporary mental anguish, and therefore incompetence, one could understand why it would be excusable, but not laudable. The fact that it was lauded suggests that incompetence was not considered a factor.

If a suicide was considered inexcusable, the person who committed the act was dishonored and denied certain burial rites, but at no time have the survivors been subject to criticism or dishonor.[7]

The Christian tradition also condemns suicide in general. During the first few centuries of Christianity, martyrdom was readily accepted. Obviously, if one fervently believes in the glory and magnificence of the hereafter, it is understandable that one would wish to go there. To remain within the stress and strain of mortal society would be irrational. It was probably because of this attitude that so many of the early Christians readily accepted death at the hands of their captors.

Possibly in order to nullify this tendency, St. Augustine (354–430 C.E.), Bishop of Hippo Regius,[8] condemned suicide on the same grounds later used by St. Thomas Aquinas,[9] who stated that

(a) every creature is inclined to resist destructive forces, therefore, suicide is against nature;

(b) man belongs to society and suicide deprives the community of what is rightfully theirs;

(c) suicide usurps the right of God, who has dominion over life and death; therefore, it is an affront to God.

Aquinas subsequently stated that, "[It] is the most fateful of sins because it cannot be repented on."[10] As a result, Catholicism views suicide as a cardinal sin unless it is committed when mentally incompetent. Yet some holy virgins who committed suicide in defense of their virtue have been venerated as saints and martyrs.[11] Even the death of Jesus, who passively submitted to mortals, was used as an example of suicide by John Donne in 1644 in his defense of suicide.[12]

Suicide is also condemned on the assumption that it violates the divine precept in the form of the commandment "Thou shalt not kill."[13] With inexcusable suicide, Christian burial is expressly forbidden, especially for "those who, in full possession of their faculties, have killed themselves."[14] In practice, however, a letter from a psychiatrist or physician alleging temporary mental incompetency is considered adequate to allow proper burial.

In other traditions, suicide was considered a reasonable act when seen within the framework of some other religious beliefs. The Vikings believed that the Paradise of Valhalla was open only to those who died violently. This included suicide. Such death insured that one would be in God's presence.[15] Some religions even gave suicide, under certain circumstances, a sense of nobility. In the Hindu ritual of *suttee*, the wife of the deceased commits suicide on her husband's funeral pyre.

SOCIAL ATTITUDES TOWARD SUICIDE

Historically, social attitudes toward suicide have covered an enormous spectrum, ranging from extreme permissiveness with actual assistance to suicide, to considering suicide an act to be condemned, degraded, feared, and hated. Some groups see it as an act to be supported and applauded, while others consider it an abomination against both God and the state. Some consider it rational, altruistic, and noble, while others consider it irrational and self-serving.

Certain societies have found the suicidal person's death frightening, and the ghost of such a person was to be feared. The body was frequently degraded, the name defamed, and the deceased became a symbol of derision and scorn.

Those who have failed in the suicide attempt have been either tortured to death or forced to receive medical care. They have been treated with scorn by some and with compassion and care by others. Independent of, but certainly supported by, religious belief and superstitions, suicide was punishable in England and Europe well into the nineteenth century not only by degradation of the body, but by confiscation of all titles and properties, since people were considered the property of the state and therefore not free to take their own lives.[16]

Many diverse societies, ancient and contemporary, primitive and sophisticated, have respected and approved of suicide.

Permissiveness, including offering assistance to suicides was within the mores of Marseilles, France, and Ceos, Greece,[17] where citizens who wished to be released from life's anguish could request permission to commit suicide from the city's officials and, if granted, receive the necessary poison. Suicide was also an acceptable alternative in some societies when life lost much of its meaning or when one's sense of worth was destroyed. Slaves frequently preferred suicide to lifelong slavery or personal degradation. This led to the mass suicide at Masada. The Epicureans and Stoics of Greece chose death when life was devoid of pleasure.[18] It was also an alternative to torture and execution (as in the suicide of King Saul[19]) or to prevent harm to one's own people, as when captured spies with vital information would kill themselves.

In some societies suicide of the elderly has been accepted when ecological factors made it difficult for the younger members of the family or group to survive. This was especially true among the more nomadic people such as the Eskimos and Scythians, the ancient people of Iran. Among the Eskimos, to assist an elderly parent to achieve death was a child's obligation, an act of supreme respect.

The attitudes within our own society are inconsistent and at times irrational. We go so far as to rigorously prevent the suicide of persons who are to be executed. We prefer to kill them rather than permit them to kill themselves. Religion, superstition, remnants of the slave state psychology, and personal fears about death are the most pertinent factors in our distorted approach toward the competent individual who performs this most final of acts.

LEGAL ASPECTS

Suicide is not a crime in any of our states, while assisting a suicide is punishable in several states. It is important at this time to dispel one commonly held misconception: that the preservation of life is a vital state interest. The state's interest is in the preservation of free choice of the individual and the prevention of harm to others. It is the individual's right of free choice that leads to the desire to live, which must therefore be respected, or the desire to die, which should be equally respected. Physicians are not infrequently faced with the request to help someone who is terminally ill to die. This is easier said than done. To do so, even secretly, places the doctor in jeopardy.

AN APPROACH TO SUICIDE

Let us see if we can establish a systematic approach to the question of suicide using our proposed ethical guidelines. Of the four factors to be considered in suicide, the right of self-determination and beneficence are the major factors to be balanced. The factors of common good and nonmaleficence become relatively insignificant in this discussion. Let us see how self-determination and beneficence apply to the various categories of individuals who might commit suicide.

The Incompetent Person

Let us first consider minors and temporarily incompetent adults. We could reason that these individuals are immature or emotionally incompetent, or both, and are therefore con-

sidered not capable of making a sound decision. This would
lead to a decision to prevent any suicide attempt. In regard
to the adult, the public does not know that the person may
not be helped by either psychological or social support. Most
suicides and attempted suicides are the result of temporary
irrational states—most often depression. This warrants interference under the factor of beneficence. We may reasonably
assume that when a rational state has been restored, the
person would appreciate the fact that the suicide had been
prevented.

Next there are the permanently and mentally severely
incompetent persons. The fundamental question to be asked
here is: What would that person's decision be if fully aware
of the permanent nature of the tragic condition? The observer
is placed in the position of making a "substituted judgment."
Assuming that if the individual were fully aware and competent, he or she would not wish to live in a permanent,
severely incompetent state, then we must respect that decision. If in doubt, then we are obligated, under the factor
of benevolence, to try to prevent the act. If we are aware
of the severity and permanence of the illness, we should not
prevent or treat effects of the action if reasonable "substituted
judgment" would agree with the correctness of the act. The
individual's right of free choice would have to be respected.

The Competent Person

We now come to a category where physicians may be of
help to patients. We should, under the factor of benevolence,
try to dissuade those rational people who attempt suicide
in order to alert society to social inequities from that type
of protest, but we have no moral right to use force to stop
their attempt. Beneficence cannot be *imposed* upon a competent person. The second group of rational people who wish
to commit suicide desire to be released from life's physical
or mental anguish. Under the doctrine of beneficence, society

must do everything in its power to encourage the person to live, to improve the person's emotional state through psychotherapy, and to reduce pain and discomfort. On a broader scale, this also means improving whatever social ills exist that may be factors leading to the decision. A ready acceptance of suicide would be an abrogation of our obligation to help the elderly, or the weak and lonely individual who feels unwanted and detached from society. But if the decision to commit suicide is based upon a rational evaluation that life in a hopeless state of anguish is not worth maintaining, then, as a general principle, society does not have the right to negate that person's freedom of choice.

Case Study

A sixty-eight-year-old male attempted suicide by driving his car into a telephone pole. In the emergency room, he refused to give consent for surgery to control a severe internal hemorrhage. He wanted to die. A few weeks earlier he had been diagnosed as having cancer of the tongue. Surgery to remove the tongue had been refused. He stated that he had had a good professional and personal life and now wished to end it.[20]

The physicians were faced with a dilemma. Should they respect the patient's refusal of life-saving surgery? Opposition to his refusal could be based on the assumption that the patient was incompetent. A substituted judgment could then be made by asking the following question: "What would I not want done to me if I were in the same position?" More specifically, "What would the patient not want done to him if he were competent?" This question was answered in a way that resulted in treatment.

The only other basis for treatment without consent would be to assume that the patient's death, under these circumstances, would cause undue harm to others. It is quite reasonable to assume that at the age of sixty-eight the "harm" in the form of family sadness that may result from his death was not sufficient to negate his free choice, especially in view of the potential distress for the patient and concomitant sorrow within the family as his disease progressed along a very unpleasant road to death. Therefore, the physicians had to balance the patient's right of free choice against the factor of beneficence, which can only be forcibly invoked if there is an element of incompetency.

Although the patient spoke rationally, it was assumed that the suicide attempt was performed while under an intolerable emotional burden. There was also the impression that the attempt was half-hearted, since the method used to commit suicide was certainly not one that usually leads to death. Therefore, an assumption was made that the patient was temporarily incompetent and might possibly be helped with psychotherapy. With this assumption, beneficence was warranted to abridge freedom of choice in order for the patient to receive psychiatric care.

On the other hand, it would have been just as reasonable to assume that since surgery was refused after suicide had been attempted, and since the patient appeared rational, his right of self-determination is too precious to be negated by the vague possibility that he acted during a period of relative incompetence.

This is a grey area where one may arrive at two different decisions, each with relatively adequate reason.

There are times when the desire to die is rational and wise. It is during those times that the physician may reasonably be expected to help the patient. Although doctors may be criticized for doing so, it is not uncommon for physicians to prescribe a larger number of sedatives than usual with full understanding of how they may be used. In reality the vast majority of patients who have access to such medication, know how to use it, and have good reason to use it, never take advantage of the opportunity. But there are patients who deserve more specific help. In those who are hopelessly ill nature frequently replaces fear with a sensibility that welcomes death. In 1961, Percy C. Bridgman, a Nobel laureate in physics who was dying of cancer, shot himself at the age of eighty. He left this final note:

> It isn't decent for society to make a man do this thing to himself. Probably this is the last day I will be able to do it myself.[21]

Was it warranted, asks fellow Nobel laureate Max Delbruck, that

> because of society's emphasis on the prolongation of life at all costs, he had to end his own life in a lonely and agonizing way? Both his family and his physician should have given him the opportunity to take his own life in a dignified way.[22]

Death-dealing medication left by the bedside of a dying person can be a blessing to one in this kind of need. At times, death may be a welcome release from an untenable life, a release from agony to be sought, not avoided. This is not an issue of holding life less precious, but of considering death less terrifying. When doctors or society impose decisions that thwart someone's reasonable act of suicide, we must be cognizant of the role that our own personal fear of death may play and appreciate the fact that this fear is often absent in the hopelessly ill.

Recently, material has been published on how to commit suicide gracefully.[23] Such public information may produce more harm than good. A "how to do it" manual of techniques may be unwisely used by temporarily depressed children and adults. But I fully understand the motivation of the author who is dedicated to helping those who need help and at the same time frustrated that the political climate has been slow in responding to this need. It may be much more prudent to place the responsibility for solving this problem upon the medical profession in conjunction with the patient's family.

There has been in recent years much discussion concerning the passage of laws authorizing physicians to assist dying or near-dying patients who wish to hasten their own deaths. This seems a reasonable approach since the obligation of the physician is to help patients. But laws, however well motivated, in their striving to include all variables, tend to complicate and confuse issues and frequently disturb helpful and wise patterns of behavior.

Many physicians traditionally have supplied dying patients who have requested help enough medication to end their lives if taken all at once. Some patients slowly accumulate medication to be able to take an overdose if they so desire. These patients are informed and well aware of the effect of such action, but it is rare that they take advantage of the opportunity. The discussions concerning these most intimate thoughts and desires of a dying patient should not be tampered with. Such discussions and decisions should remain within the intimate rapport among patient, doctor, and family. Physicians entrusted with the wisdom and judgment to treat patients with dangerous drugs, as all drugs are, and to invade the heart and even enter the brain of a person in order to prolong life should certainly be entrusted with the much less complicated problems of managing an already dying patient. The actions of Jack Kevorkian[24] are of interest. His basic premise to assist those in need to end life is commendable, but the judgment used in the selection of cases is highly questionable. Rather than pass laws to speak to this problem, I believe that those states with statutes that consider assisted suicide a crime should annul the statutes. If that is done and if physicians appreciate that their role is to help patients, which is broader than the idea that their role is only to prolong life, why enact laws making something legal that is already not illegal and thereby disturb helpful and wise behavior patterns? To assist a patient who wishes to end the agony of their dying hours or days is in every sense fulfilling the physician's obligation to help his or her patient. This assistance has been and still is part of medicine.

Many physicians will feel very uneasy acceding to their patient's request. Although it may be reasonable and morally correct to assist a patient to die, it is contrary to all medical tradition, their training, and the whole ambience of their existence, which has been directed toward the preservation of life. Religious training may absolutely forbid such assistance. Their own psyche may not allow them to accept the thought that they were instrumental in helping a patient to die. One cannot fault any of these reasons. One can only fault a physician who cannot comply with the request for not transferring the patient to a different doctor's care.

SUICIDE VERSUS CAPITAL PUNISHMENT

There will probably be a gradual increase in executions across the United States. States that formerly banned capital punishment are now rethinking the issue. Regardless of whether or not one is an advocate of capital punishment, if it becomes the law of the land, there is need to reevaluate our attitude toward this form of punishment. There appears to be an understandable but undesirable element of revenge inherent in certain aspects of criminal punishment. This factor becomes most apparent during discussions about capital punishment.

At the present time, extreme measures are enforced to prevent condemned prison inmates from committing suicide. Such efforts are not motivated by societal benevolence, as when we prevent the suicide of a depressed youngster or adult, but rather are based upon a semiconscious, if not conscious, desire to avoid losing the opportunity for revenge. In the face of certain crimes, our anger is such that when a condemned prisoner commits suicide, it is looked upon as cheating society of its just and proper due. Death does not appear to be an adequate punishment unless it is exercised by society and observed by spectators.

It would appear that a reevaluation of our attitude about suicide among prisoners is in order. One may postulate that the philosophy preventing suicide among condemned prisoners is part of the punishment—the removal of the right to determine the way they must die, to choose between execution and suicide.

Some will ask: Why not allow the child molester or rapist to commit suicide if the person so desires? It is obvious that the condemned inmate has that right, as does any other citizen.

It is in the name of societal benevolence, the thrust to protect the weak and the innocent, that we prevent people from committing suicide, but a criminal loses the right to society's benevolence in proportion to the degree of the crime.

The individual who has killed another person without good reason, the child molester, the rapist, and other such criminals, must be considered least qualified for society's benevolence. Suicide under such circumstances should not be prevented. If such criminals desire to die, regardless of the stressful circumstances, their freedom of choice outweighs the residual amount of state beneficence due them. Such a prisoner should not only be permitted to commit suicide, he or she should be given an opportunity to do so. It is strange that our society is ready to imprison for life, hang, electrocute, poison with gas, or shoot a criminal but does not permit the condemned criminal to use a pill to die. This attitude seems barbaric unless we wish to accept that we are a vengeful society.

We should seriously consider modifying our laws to

eliminate the present policies that actively prevent suicide among such prisoners. We should not only permit their suicide but enable them to end their lives by allowing access to the proper medication under rigid control.

The Greek philosopher Socrates and the Roman Seneca were both given the privilege of suicide. If persons are to be executed, it would be preferable for them to kill themselves rather than impose that burden on society. To allow prisoners to commit suicide, with or without assistance, does not necessarily mean that they will mimic Socrates, but at least we should permit them to do so. To the extent that suicide for the condemned will be permitted, society will be less debased.

NOTES

1. *The American Heritage Dictionary of the English Language,* William Morris, ed. (Boston: Houghton Mifflin Company, 1979).

2. Genesis 9:6, 9:5.

3. Ahitophel, 2 Samuel 17:23; Saul, 1 Samuel 31:3-5; Saul's armor bearer, 1 Samuel 31:5; Abimelech, Judges 9:54; Zimri, I Kings 16:18; Samson, Judges 16:30.

4. Harm Cohen, "Suicide in Jewish Legal and Religious Tradition," *Journal of Mental Health and Society* 3 (1976): 129.

5. Ibid., p. 134.

6. Ibid., p.133.

7. Ibid., p. 136.

8. St. Augustine, *Select Letters with an English Translation,* by J. H. Baxter (New York: Putnam's Sons, 1930), p. 291, section 39:5.

9. *The Summa Theologica of St. Thomas Aquinas,* Vol. 2 (New York: Benzinger Brothers, Inc., 1947), p. 1469, Question 64, Article 5.

10. Ibid., p. 1469.

11. Hd. Most Rev. William J. McDonald, D.D., Ph.D., ed., *New Catholic Encyclopedia,* Vol. 13 (New York: McGraw Hill Book Company, n.d.), p. 782.

12. John Donne, *Biathanatos,* Garland English Texts No. 1, Michael Rudick and M. Pabst Battin, eds. (New York: Garland Publishers Inc., 1982), pp. LXXX, 172-74, 268, Part I, Distinction 3.

13. St. Augustine, *Selected Letters*.

14. McDonald, *New Catholic Encyclopedia*, Vol. 2, p. 897.

15. A. Alverez, *The Savage God* (New York: Random House, 1972), p. 46.

16. Ibid., p. 47.

17. Ibid., p. 61.

18. Ibid., p. 60.

19. 1 Samuel 31:3–5.

20. M. Jellinek, R. Brandt, and R. Litman, "A Suicide Attempt and Emergency Room Ethics," *Hastings Center Report* (August 1979): 12–13.

21. Max Delbruck, "Education for Suicide," *Prism* (November 1974): 50.

22. Ibid.

23. Derek Humphry, *Final Exit: The Practicalities of Self-Deliverance and Assisted Suicide for the Dying* (Eugene, Ore.: The Hemlock Society, 1991).

24. Jack Kevorkian, *Prescription: Medicide: The Goodness of Planned Death* (Buffalo, N.Y.: Prometheus Books, 1991).

6

Abortion

Abortion is an ancient and controversial issue that will remain with us as long as women continue to conceive. It includes the human tragedy of parental anguish and the death of a living embryo. As a result it has become a highly charged issue, a political football associated with half truths, distorted truths, and vitriolic accusations.

I shall attempt to outline the basic arguments for and against abortion, and to assess their validity from the standpoint of the ethical stance discussed in chapter 1. In this discussion all four factors—autonomy, nonmaleficence, common good, and beneficence—are of importance.

From the outset, I would like to discuss one word that has become prominent in this controversy, namely, "murder." Regardless whether one is anti-abortion or pro-choice, limited or otherwise, use of the term "murder" is inappropriate. We may speak of killing the conceptus, the embryo, or the fetus, but we cannot speak of murder. Murder is to kill with malice or evil intent. In other words, murder demonstrates the presence of a callous, insensitive feeling toward the person harmed. A murderer is rarely, if ever, respectful of human life, although the murderer may later have a sense of guilt and a sense of remorse. This is not at all the case for a woman or teenager who has an abortion. Although it occurs, it is unusual that a woman would have a feeling of malice toward the conceptus or fetus.

Almost all abortions are to some degree a source of regret, anguish, distress, and sorrow. It is inaccurate to assume that a woman contemplating abortion does not have respect for fetal life, is insensitive to the moral dilemma she faces, or that the thirteen-year-old child who has been raped and is to have an abortion is a murderer. Respect for life is usually not part of the psyche of a murderer. When "murder" is used during a discussion of abortion it arouses emotions which inhibit reasoned discourse. The abortion debate does not need added emotion. I am discussing murder and malice as they are generally understood and not as a technical term used in law.

There are six major arguments against abortion.

1. Fetal life is sacred. The sanctity of life has been stressed by religious segments of society. It implies a hallowed state from God. But the emphasis upon sanctity is possibly due to the strong Christian stance that unless the infant or newborn can be baptized, it may be condemned to hell;

2. The possible dehumanizing influence upon society if abortion is permitted;

3. The state's compelling interest in preserving life;

4. The possible unwarranted and dangerous extrapolation of applying the reasons for abortion to the newborn and even to the older child and adult—an extrapolation that could lead to an acceptance of homicide of the defective newborn child or adult (a concept well expressed by Ramsey[1]);

5. The problem of creating a category that discriminates life according to circumstances; and

6. The idea that the conceptus is a person with a right to life.

Professor Jay Katz suggests that there may be an underlying motive, applicable to many anti-abortionists, which has remained unspoken. Those who are unfortunate enough to feel or be told that they were unwanted, or disliked during early family turmoil, may unconsciously be striking back at their parents by condemning abortion, which to them strongly symbolizes the "not being wanted" concept. To approve abortion may be unconsciously sensed as affirming the right of their parents to have disliked or not wanted them.[2]

The first argument, that life is sacred, cannot be accepted simply because it is based on religious dogma and we are discussing ethical approaches in a secular framework, as previously described. This does not mean that life is not precious and awesome, but only that the theological doctrine that ties life to a God concept must be set aside if we are to discuss this within a secular framework. "Sanctity" implies "sanctified by God." A large segment of anti-abortionists use this concept as the basis for opposing abortion except possibly to save the life of a mother. In many respects the attempt to impose a concept derived from religious dogma upon a secular society reflects a remarkable disrespect for our traditional separation of church and state. But the sanctity-of-life concept has been of value. It has served to temper a detached or mechanical approach to decision making. It asks for a more intense respect for life. This can only intensify our sense of caution.

The second argument, that abortion may have a dehumanizing influence, is very questionable in view of the history of war, hatred, bigotry, poverty, and famine in our world. It seems far-fetched to assume that sanctioning abortion, which would appear like a blink in this history, would have a significant dehumanizing effect upon society and therefore be contrary to the common good. The modern Chinese, who strongly advocate abortions for control of population, do not appear to be any more dehumanized than prior regimes in which the starvation of millions was a yearly event. Daniel Callahan also expresses his doubt about any significant detriment to the common good resulting from legalized abortion: "Whatever one may think of the morality of abortion, it cannot be established that it poses a clear and present danger to the common good."[3]

The third point, compelling state interest, is based on a misconception of fundamental constitutional provisions. The state's "compelling interest," its primary interest regarding life, is not the preservation of life but the preservation of the more fundamental right of self-determination: freedom of choice. It is this right of free choice that leads to the preservation of life. *A person's right to life is derived from the decision of that person to live.* In regard to incompetent people, which includes minor children, the state has an obligation under beneficence to protect and nourish such people and to foster actions that will be best for them. If that means to preserve life, very well, but that is different than the "state's compelling interest to preserve life." Rather, its compelling interest is to help people. What is meant by "help" will vary with each situation. It need not necessarily be equated with the preservation of life.

The fourth argument against abortion is that if there is adequate reason to abort, that same reason could be used to justify infanticide. The argument is therefore not so much against abortion per se but against abortion as the beginning of a slippery slope to presumably unwarranted actions after birth. This problem will be discussed in chapter 8, on euthanasia.

The fifth argument addresses the danger of creating a category of life that may be discriminated against according to circumstances. This is very similar to the fourth point. It raises the specter of wholesale euthanasia for retarded older children and adults. This, too, will be discussed later.

This leads to the sixth and possibly the most pertinent argument: that the conceptus is a person and has the same rights as any other person. The concept of personhood or humanhood has not been clearly defined in spite of an extensive literature that has attempted to do so.[4-5] It is my impression that the arguments placing personhood at the time of conception, or asserting that the attributes of personhood (and therefore personhood itself) depend upon factors such as the conceptus's awareness of its own existence, intellectual development, the capacity to form relationships, or social independence, are all attempts to validate a preconceived position regarding the rightness or wrongness of abortion. It is quite a matter of personal preference whether one considers the conceptus, the seven-month-old fetus, or the two-year-old child as a legal person. The argument can be made that the conceptus is a person since it can receive property willed to it, but property can also be willed to a bird.

*   *   *

Much of the abortion debate revolves around the issue of personhood, which can never be resolved through reason alone. Let us, for the sake of discussion, accept the conceptus as a person and avoid the situation where someone not fully developed or not quite normal may be considered a nonperson. Where does acceptance of this stance, so strongly suggested by certain theological groups, lead us?

If we accept the premise that the conceptus is a person from the first second of its formation, we must grant that person all the rights and privileges and full respect due the incompetent or competent adult or the minor child. Therefore, the mere fact that it is not fully developed and is incompetent should not in any way denigrate its rights as a full citizen.

Those who oppose abortion accept this concept and therefore believe that the competing claims between an embryo's right to life and a potential mother's right to privacy or right of free choice are not equal in weight. In other words, certain death of a person deserves more consideration than possible harm or inconvenience to another. On the surface this appears to be a very cogent argument against abortion, but when the problem of abortion is posed in this manner it obscures the more fundamental issue that must be uncovered before a dispassionate decision can be made—human rights and human dignity.

What is this dignity of humanhood and personhood granted the conceptus? This dignity was well expressed by Massachusetts Justice J. Liacos in the Saikewicz case:

> The principles of equality and respect . . . must extend to the case of an incompetent, as well as a competent patient because the value of human dignity extends to both. . . .
>
> To presume that the incompetent person must always be subjected to what many rational and intelligent persons may decline is to downgrade the status of the incompetent person by placing a lesser value on his intrinsic human worth and vitality.[6]

If we respect this concept and if we accept the conceptus and fetus as people, we must grant them this right of self-determination. To abort or not to abort without full consideration of the developing embryo's right to choose is to place a lesser value on its "intrinsic human worth" and to negate its human dignity. To avoid this pitfall, "substituted judgment" must be made, a judgment that, as expressed by Justice Liacos, "would be made by the incompetent person, if that person were competent."[7] We must therefore ask what the conceptus would wish to do if able to express his or her desire. It is not pertinent what you or I might choose but only what the incompetent in question would choose, regardless whether it be a conceptus or an adult in a coma.*

---

*The reasoning for the use of substituted judgment instead of the "best interests" doctrine has been discussed in chapter 4.

Within this line of reasoning, since life or death of a person (the conceptus) is at stake, the wishes of the conceptus assume a primary position and the desires of the mother or father become secondary. This holds true unless the life of the fetus is pitted against the life of the mother. Such situations are very rare.

Who is to make that substituted judgment for the developing human? Can it be made by family and physician, or must it go through due process in court? Can parents, physicians, or a judge place themselves in that position? Can we ever be certain of the answer? We can appreciate the dilemma, yet a decision *must* be made. If not, a decision is automatically made (i.e., the birth occurs) without due regard and respect for what that particular incompetent human may desire.

For the moment we shall put aside the problem of who should make a substituted judgment for a developing conceptus and discuss the decision-making process itself. What are the questions that the conceptus would need to consider in order to reach a decision? There are many questions, to be sure, but at minimum they include nine to be answered with the realization that human relationships have not yet begun.

1. What is the quality of its future mental state?

2. What is the quality of its future physical state?

3. Will it be wanted?

4. Will it be abused?

5. Will it live a normal life span?

6. Will its life be one of physical or mental anguish?

7. Will it suffer hunger and malnourishment?

8. Will it be a source of anguish for its parents?

9. Will it live at home or in an institution?

After due consideration of at *least* these nine factors, whoever is to make the substituted judgment must then ask what that conceptus would wish to have done.

Since we can determine the presence of over 1,600 diseases during the first trimester of pregnancy, let us discuss the decision making for a conceptus with a specific illness that is detectable in the early stages of development.

Tay-Sachs disease is an incurable genetic disorder characterized by progressive blindness, severe mental deterioration and death usually by the age of six. This is obviously an extreme case. If it is known that the embryo is suffering from Tay-Sachs disease and the parents are considering abortion, a "substituted judgment" must be made for the embryo independent of the parents' wishes. Would that specific embryo, if aware of the circumstances, wish to be aborted, or would it wish to continue its path toward birth? What would that embryonic person, who we must assume would desire to be an intelligent, competent adult, say if it were able to express an opinion? Would it demand to continue toward birth, live its short, horribly defective life, and impose anguish and heartache upon its parents during its life span and forever in their minds? Or would it demand to be aborted? What would be the decision?

The framework used to make such decisions is what the average person, free of religious constraints, or able to be objective despite religious beliefs, would decide if transposed into that fetal state and condition. Would such a frame of reference lead to an absolutely reliable answer? Certainly not! We can only make a reasonable judgment. In the case of Tay-Sachs disease most people would opt for abortion. It would therefore appear reasonable to assume that, in such terrible circumstances, a conceptus, through substituted judgment, would prefer to be aborted rather than to die soon after birth and bring such anguish upon its parents.

Although it is reasonable to assume that the conceptus would wish to be aborted if tragically ill, there is a great distance, with infinite gradations, between the devastation of Tay-Sachs disease and a perfectly normal existence with normal physical and mental capabilities. Can we so easily assume that a healthy conceptus would opt for abortion simply because a wealthy woman of thirty-eight does not wish to be bothered by a new child? Would that not be considered a trivial reason for abortion from the embryo's point of view?

Within this approach, when we move from the extremes of tragedy whereby substituted judgment, reasonably and without significant question, would warrant abortion, to trivial inconvenience, the certainty of decision making becomes less clear and more tenuous. We move into a grey area where rigidity and dogmatic positions become inappropriate and decision making becomes more arduous. When abortion is proposed to avoid trivial inconvenience, we reach a point where it is reasonable to assume that "substituted judgment" for the conceptus would be to continue its path toward birth. The assumption may be made that even if it is unwanted by its real parents, it could be loved and wanted by childless couples.

Even though it is theoretically possible that the conceptus would reply in the negative if asked whether it would prefer to be born if the mother does not want it, the preponderance of weight is probably in favor of preservation of life.

There can be no sharp line drawn to determine the point when abortion is or is not warranted from the conceptus's point of view. In this grey area of decision making there can be legitimate differences of opinion even though the conceptus is granted the right of personhood. Therefore a dogmatic stance by either side, which would lead one to *impose* views upon another, is unacceptable.

Let us now look at the issue from a different point of view. If we do not look at the conceptus and embryo as a person but only as an organism with potential for human qualities, dogmatic opposition to abortion becomes unreasonable and unwarranted compared with a woman's right of privacy and self-determination.

All other arguments for abortion, all other factors used to support the mother's right to decide, are relatively secondary. Such factors are not really necessary, since the mother's right to decide would need no support.

The arguments supporting pro-choice are based on beneficence toward the potential mother as well as the fetus, respect for the woman's right of self-determination and privacy, and concern for the common good of society. They tend to support reasons for abortion and therefore reasons for retaining laws that permit safe and legal abortions. The following concepts are commonly used.

1. Regardless whether abortion is legal and safe or illegal and unsafe, hundreds of thousands of women will seek abortion. When abortion was illegal the mortality and morbidity rate—the incidence of death, sickness and permanent disability—was very high. Almost 30 percent of all maternal deaths were due to illegal abortions.[8] The prevention of these tragedies should be a goal of society.

2. To make abortions illegal will tend to harm the poor. The wealthy can travel to obtain a safe and legal abortion. The young and the poor will suffer. They will seek an illegal abortion and be subject to a high rate of complications and death.

3. The fetus is a threatening entity, since it is more dangerous to give birth than it is to have an abortion. It is therefore not a harmless organism. It is a physical threat to the health and life of the mother. Many women are seriously ill and in danger of losing their life during pregnancy and childbirth. The mortality from childbirth is sixteen times greater than the mortality from a legal abortion.

4. Genetic defects account for approximately 25 percent of newborn deaths. Many of these tragedies facing young parents can be avoided through genetic counseling and studies. The emotional trauma in such situations is immense and the psychological scars can persist for years.

5. Acquired immunodeficiency syndrome is undoubtedly going to become more prevalent. Mothers with AIDS may transmit the disease to the newborn. Many of these newborns will die within several years. This tragedy could be avoided by testing pregnant women and by elective abortions.

6. Teenage, unwed mothers tend to drop out of school and thereby fail to fulfill their intellectual potential. This group is frequently condemned to poverty and subsequently becomes a significant economic burden upon society.

7. The psychological impact upon a young teenager faced with the burden of motherhood can be extremely destructive.

8. The psychological harm to a mother who has given up her newborn for adoption is much greater than the psychological harm to the woman who has an abortion. Many anti-abortionists seem to accept the reality of psychological harm, yet they make their own distinctions about how much harm is enough to warrant an abortion. Many anti-abortionists approve of abortion for the twelve-year-old rape victim so that she does not suffer all the physical and psychological trauma childbirth may bring; they also approve of abortion for the child who becomes pregnant as a result of incest, but yet they remain opposed to abortion in the case of a potential mother who would be suicidal with a newborn or when faced with

the agony of a pregnant mother whose children are already starving or severely malnourished.

9. The emotional trauma to a woman who is forced to continue an unwanted pregnancy with a normal fetus is markedly compounded for the woman carrying a fetus which she knows would develop into a handicapped child. We must also consider the tremendous emotional harm to siblings and parents faced with a newborn who is severely handicapped. Many families are destroyed under these circumstances.

10. When abortion is denied, the psychological and sociological problems facing the unwanted child are destructive. These children have a higher rate of juvenile delinquency, drug abuse, and crime. The parents suffer, the children suffer, and society suffers.

11. The cost to our nation if abortions were unavailable would be an additional $12 billion per year. Fifty percent of abortions involve teenagers. The present welfare expense for teenage mothers and their children is $18 billion per year. This would probably climb to approximately $30 billion per year.[9] There is no reason for society to be burdened with this additional undesirable expense.

12. Until a good contraceptive program is found, abortion is a necessary adjunct for family planning. Population control is a world problem. Starvation and malnutrition are devastating in many areas of the world. For children to be brought into the world only to die of hunger or to live a malnourished life is an unwarranted and unnecessary evil. If abortions were to stop this world problem would become even more agonizing. Aside from the Catholic Church, which has been insensitive to this problem, the anti-abortionists see the issue only in local terms, related to

our relatively affluent society in the United States. They appear unaware of the compounding world tragedies that would unfold if abortions worldwide were to cease.

13. The population demands upon our environment are a very significant factor underlying the destruction of Earth's biomass and pollution of our air and waters.

The approach accepted by the United States Supreme Court in the *Roe* v. *Wade* decision (1973) was that the developing organism was not considered a legal person with constitutional rights that the state has an obligation to protect. Therefore the fetus was declared not to have the rights and privileges of legal personhood until birth. However, the state's interest increases with time, beginning at the third trimester of pregnancy, at which time the fetus has reached the stage of natural viability. Prior to this time, abortion is only subject to the potential mother's right to self-determination. This right, in conjunction with her right of privacy, would obviously be more important than the "rights" of a nonperson developing organism within her body. The court stated that, "The right of privacy . . . is broad enough to encompass a woman's decision whether or not to terminate her pregnancy."[10]

If abortion were to be unavailable, who would accept responsibility for the unwanted newborn? If institutionalization is necessary, must society be forced to supply funds for lifelong care? Should the taxpayer be forced to support a seriously handicapped unwanted child in an institution for the rest of its life? It is of interest to note that most of those who are strongly anti-abortion—who vigorously demonstrate, protest, and even use violence—are not seen demonstrating for the greater economic aid needed to *support* that life adequately, nor do they individually offer to care for an unwanted handicapped child. As Churchill and Simon so aptly state,

> Their advocacy for the fetus is grounded in a self-serving and fragmented notion of life. Fetal life is valued and protected but the obligation to support the newborn, adolescent or adult life is absent. A logic that sees more obligations to life *in utero* but fails to accept responsibility for the quality of life *extra-uterum* is myopic . . . it is easy to fight for fetal life if it requires none of one's own resources to maintain that life later. This isolation of the right to life is frightening and profoundly anti-social.[11]

If we accept abortion in cases of rape or incest, we are placing relative values on the degree of danger to potential mothers' psychological and physical health as criteria for abortion. If so, are we also permitted to place relative values related to physical health or the state of development of the uterine contents? What is the value of a conceptus as compared to the value of the seven-month-old fetus? If the value is less in the first trimester, is abortion warranted since maternal life is threatened by childbirth? If the value is less, is self-defense a valid reason for abortion? Some very sensitive and socially responsible people may ask an even more probing question. What makes life at the prebonding, nonrelational period valuable or precious? Have we arbitrarily placed such value judgments on a fertilized egg in order to satisfy preconceived ideas peculiar to our particular culture?

If abortion is absolutely condemned, should not contraceptive methods such as the IUD (intrauterine device) be condemned as well? The IUD prevents the conceptus from adhering to the wall of the uterus. This is tantamount to putting grease on the ledge of a window so that a child holding on for dear life will fall. If we do not condemn IUDs, is there any significant difference between preventing a conceptus from holding on and scraping it off the wall of the uterus after implantation has taken place? Although we may draw such a line, is it not arbitrary?

There are several other aspects to this problem. Can the conceptus, as a person, demand through substituted judgment to be aborted? Can a fetus developing in the body of a devout Catholic woman demand, through reasonable substituted judgment, that the woman submit to an abortion against her will, or, for that matter, demand that the physician perform an abortion?

Can a conceptus developing in a thirty-five-year-old woman demand, through substituted judgment, that genetic studies be performed to be certain that enough data is available for proper decision making? This may lead to abortion or reveal the need for intrauterine treatment, or treatment to be instituted immediately after birth. Parents have sued physicians and laboratories for lack of information or misinformation that prevented them from reaching a decision that would have reasonably led to an abortion of the fetus. Such legal actions have been termed "wrongful birth" suits. The basis for such action is the immense (often devastating) physical, economic, and psychological burden imposed upon the parents and family of a seriously damaged newborn.

If reasonable substituted judgment is ignored and flaunted and a fetus is forced to be born into a state of physical and mental anguish when it reasonably would not have wished to have been born, would that person, when it is an adult, have the right to sue and seek compensation against parents who wrongfully disobeyed its right of self-determination? Legal actions in a similar vein by a child or on behalf of a child are termed "wrongful life" actions. This concept refers to the claim against a physician or laboratory by a person (or through a surrogate if incompetent) that they would have preferred to have been aborted rather than to have been born. Analysis of the legal and philosophical ramifications of these two issues are well discussed by Elias and Annas,[12] Capron,[13] and Steinbock.[14]

From the point of view of respect for autonomy and non-maleficence and for consistency in application it is apparent that the wrongful birth and wrongful life legal actions are reasonably based. In principle everyone has a right to information that could affect decisions regarding a medical situation. When potential parents seek medical advice regarding actual pregnancy they have the right to know all possible complications and side effects of the pregnancy, as well as all factors pertinent to the health of the fetus. This is the basis for informed consent. It is irrelevant what their decision would be. The decision itself is not what is crucial. It is only relevant that they *have the right* to make a decision based upon data that they *have a right* to expect from their attending physician. Physicians are quite properly expected to inform pregnant women about congenital and genetic problems as part of the informed consent necessary to manage the state of pregnancy.

Where should the power to decide lie in the management of pregnancy? If we assume that society has a right to dictate what a woman must do with her conceptus, does society also have a right to decide what a woman must do with her ova or a man with his sperm? Are these not living organisms with human potential? Should anyone other than potential parents have a right to decide whether a woman should or should not become pregnant, the right to the management of their ova and sperm? If pregnancy occurs, would not the most reasonable parties to decide regarding the management of the pregnancy still be the parents, regardless of whether or not the conceptus is considered a person? Are not the potential parents (or parent) in as good, if not a better position, to make a decision as any other member of society? Medical consultation and advice would obviously be involved.

It seems quite arbitrary to remove parental control of a sperm and ovum that have just been joined together because a new label of personhood may have been placed upon that union. Societal interference in such a personal matter is somewhat suggestive of the time when the use of contraception was considered a crime. Religious self-righteousness denied husbands and wives control over their own sperm and ovum. This astounding invasion of privacy remained a law in the state of Connecticut until it was declared unconstitutional by the United States Supreme Court in the *Griswold* case.[15] Autonomy and its byproduct, privacy, were at stake. Could we be facing a resurgence of such restrictive attitudes as a result of religious dictates?

At the present time in the United States, abortion is accepted on the basis of privacy of the mother until the point of *natural* viability. In other words, it does not include artificially sustained viability, such as may be theoretically possible by combining an egg and a sperm and nurturing the conceptus in a test tube or artificial womb. Natural viability refers to the growth and development of the fetus, which takes place without scientific interference.

If we accept the concept of abortion and appreciate the advent of intrauterine medical and surgical therapy to treat the fetus, then genetic screening becomes an important consideration in order to identify the fetus that may need treatment.

It appears that under the concept of beneficence as well as the common good, efforts should be made to identify and inform those individuals who are prone to transmit a significant genetic disorder to a child. Most people at high risk would appreciate knowing of their problem and would appreciate recommendations for how to avert tragedy.

If genetic screening studies reveal the existence of a seriously defective embryo, do the parents have the right to allow that birth to happen? This raises the far-reaching question of whether the parental right to give birth is unqualified. Does the *ability* to have children reflect an *unqualified right* to have children? Some societies have questioned this right when population growth has reached unbearable levels.

Under the factor of the common good, it is apparent that such an act by parents would be to the detriment of society unless they could guarantee that the product of that birth is never a burden upon society. Since parents usually die before their children and since severely damaged people, especially those severely mentally retarded, are usually a burden upon society, do parents have an inalienable right to knowingly produce such children? The right of parenthood would appear to be qualified, as all rights are. The problem would be to know where to draw the line. Although I pose the problem I do not have a comfortable answer. It would appear warranted to pass laws necessitating abortion if it were known that the damaged fetus would become a burden upon society, but I do not know how such a law could be formulated. Therefore, if such circumstances arise, abortion should at least be encouraged.

It is a sad comment that our politicians do not permit the drug RU 486 (which is replacing surgical abortion in France) to enter the United States for further study so that surgical abortions could be avoided. If made available throughout the world, it could save thousands of women from death secondary to illegally performed abortions. The religious forces that underlie the movements to abolish legal abortions, primarily the Catholic Church, are the same forces preventing the introduction of RU 486. Such actions are reminiscent of the time when these same groups made contraception illegal in the state of Connecticut. The separation between church and state is being slowly eroded.

NOTES

1. Paul Ramsey, "Feticide/Infanticide upon Request," *Religion in Life* 39 (1970): 170–86, p. 175.

2. Jay Katz, personal communication, 1990.

3. Daniel Callahan, "Abortion Decisions," in *Personal Mor-*

ality in the Problem of Abortion, Joel Feinberg, ed. (Belmont, Calif.: Wadsworth Publishing Co., 1973), p. 18.

4. H. T. Englehardt, Jr., *The Foundation of Bioethics* (New York: Oxford University Press, 1986).

5. R. M. Veatch, *A Theory of Medical Ethics* (New York: Basic Books, 1981).

6. *Superintendent of Belchertown School* v. *Joseph Saikewicz.* Mass., 370 N.B. 2d 417, p. 428.

7. Ibid., p. 431.

8. Ruth Roemer, J.D., personal communication, University of California, Los Angeles, 1990.

9. Ibid.

10. *Roe* v. *Wade,* 410 U.S. 116 (1973).

11. L. R. Churchill and J. J. Siman, "Abortion and the Rhetoric of Individual Rights," *The Hastings Center Report* 12, no. 1 (February 1982): 11.

12. S. Elias and G. J. Annas, *Reproductive Genetics and the Law* (Chicago: Year Book Medical Publishing Inc., 1987), pp. 109-20.

13. A. M. Capron, "The Wrong of Wrongful Life," in *Genetics and the Law II,* A. Milinsky and G. Annas, eds. (New York: Plenum Press, 1980), pp. 81-93.

14. B. Steinbock, "The Logical Case of Wrongful Life," *The Hastings Center Report* 16 (April 1986): 15-20.

15. *Griswold* v. *Connecticut,* 381 U.S. 479 (1965).

7

The Tragic Newborn

The following discussion will examine the problem of withholding medical care necessary to preserve life among those newborns who are seriously defective. Euthanasia, the concept of administering medication to end life immediately, will be discussed in chapter 8.

The three factors that were most relevant in the abortion discussion—nonmaleficence, beneficence, and autonomy—must also be applied when dealing with issues pertinent to newborns. The common good only becomes relevant when financial burdens are placed upon society.

The problem of the tragic newborn is poignantly stated by Professor of Child Health and Development Gordon B. Avery.

Should a severely malformed infant be resuscitated in the delivery room? . . . Should a "no code" order be written on a profoundly asphyxiated infant . . . ? Should a baby . . . who has lost his entire intestine be started on total parenteral nutrition? Is there a birth weight and gestational age below which the hope of a good outcome is too small to justify commencing intensive care? Can diminished funds justify conserving resources for those with a better

prognosis and therefore denying care to a baby with a
dismal outlook? Can a respirator be turned off when it is
supporting a baby who has massive cerebral hemorrhage
. . . but whose problems do not fulfill strict criteria of brain
death? Such situations occur regularly in every intensive
care nursery. They raise the question of whether drastic
therapy should be withheld or withdrawn in the face of
a seemingly hopeless outlook for meaningful recovery.[1]

And if so, which defective newborn should be treated? Who
should be the decision makers? Where do we draw the line
and how can we prevent the unwarranted cancellation of
treatment? Should rigid parameters be set, as in Sweden,
where neonates weighing below 750 grams (approximately
two pounds) are rarely given artificial ventilation?[2]

The management of the seriously ill newborn becomes
extremely complex for two major reasons. The first and
probably most important reason is the deeply ingrained
concept not to allow life to die. The second reason is our
difficulty in rendering a dispassionate judgment, especially
when it involves newborns and infants. Our emotional
attachments cannot be ignored. They are part of the reason
that such anguish and strong opinions are aroused when
the preservation of a newborn's life is questioned.

Natural biological thrusts have imposed upon all members of the animal kingdom, especially humans, an inherent drive to protect, nourish, and preserve the newborn. The
emotional bonding between parents and newborns becomes
very intense within a short period of time. The attitude of
the public at large is partially shaped by the transference
of our bonding with our own children to the tragic problems
that face another parent and child.

In contrast, the act of abortion is much more readily
accepted because of the relative absence of bonding during
the intrauterine stage of development. Society may be more
willing to comply with a decision leading to an abortion,

but may be very hesitant to withhold treatment from a defective newborn. This hesitancy is not necessarily based upon reason, but upon tangible anguish at the thought of a newborn's death. Associated with and inherent within this sadness is our tendency to transfer our own fears of death to the newborn.

If one denies the reasonableness of even selective abortion, and then extrapolates this attitude to the tragically endowed newborn, one would treat intensively all newborns regardless of condition and future quality of life in order to preserve that life. However, if one accepts abortion for the tragically endowed embryo, and then extrapolates that acceptance to the tragic newborn, at minimum one would avoid any effort to preserve life, and at maximum one would allow infanticide.

Both Ramsey[3] and Fletcher,[4] who stand at opposite poles on this issue, reasonably extrapolate abortion of the damaged fetus to the withholding of treatment of a newborn who would have been aborted if the tragic condition had been known. Both agree that there is no moral difference between these two acts; that it is irrational to advocate abortion during the first trimester because of a tragic illness and yet demand that the newborn with the same disease be aggressively treated in order to preserve life. As Fletcher puts it: "To have given birth innocently to a Downs case when we would not have done so if we had known the truth, does not of itself justify our extending the tragedy."[5] Ramsey's fear that this can logically be extrapolated to the older child and incompetent adult is certainly understandable, but this does not mean that such an extrapolation is beyond control. I will speak to the problem of unwarranted extrapolation later.

But fear of extrapolation is only one reason for Ramsey's opposition to the nontreatment of the seriously defective newborn. His other and perhaps most important reason is his essentially unqualified belief in the sanctity of life, his belief that life must be preserved. Ramsey therefore suggests that the only parameter for decision making at the newborn stage should be whether medical or surgical treatment is appropriate for the specific problem. If a specific abnormality can be treated it should be treated. Consideration of other factors, such as paraplegia or severe mental retardation, which are not specifically in need of treatment, would be irrelevant. Therefore, a newborn with an imperforate anus should be treated to restore anal functioning even if the newborn is mentally retarded, blind, and paraplegic. By deliberately limiting the parameters for decision making, Ramsey is then able to state: "We have no moral right to choose that some live and others die, when the medical indications for treatment are the same.[6] He attempts to reinforce this position by stating that we should use the "equality-of-life" principle rather than quality-of-life principle on the basis that the defective newborn is equally a person as the normal newborn and therefore should be treated for the same condition as an otherwise normal newborn would be treated.

But Ramsey does admit exceptions. He does accept the nontreatment of an infant with Lesch-Nyhan syndrome* or Tay-Sachs disease on the basis that "when care cannot be conveyed, it need not be extended."[7] This reason appears somewhat out of context with his usual stand and suggests that nontreatment in such cases may be warranted only because the type of illness is so severe and devastating. These exceptions weaken Ramsey's basic premise to treat what can be treated, and certainly weaken his rejection of using quality of life as a valid parameter for decision making. He should therefore accept the validity of nontreatment of defective newborns in principle and then worry about the parameters for decision making. He has decided for himself how tragic a newborn must be in order to withhold treatment but has denied that same right to others. It is not stressed often

---

*A condition recognized by mental retardation, spastic cerebral palsy, and self-mutilation.

enough that if treatment is forced upon a newborn with a tragic deficit leading to a very poor quality of life, it is the parents and their children who will have to live with that tragedy. The significance of the burden is all too often ignored.

Robert Weir rejects Ramsey's position:

> An extension of a seriously defective infant's life can represent a greater harm than does nontreatment result-ing in death. In such cases . . . to withhold treatment in order to bring about the infant's death is to do something *less harmful* to the infant than would treatment resulting in an extension of the infant's life for an indeterminate period of time . . . under such circumstances . . . the prin-ciple of nonmaleficence imposes *a duty* not to treat the child.[8]

Ramsey's concept of treating that which is treatable re-gardless of other aspects of reality is contrary to general medical practice, which considers the totality of the patient when a decision is made. To ignore looking at a newborn as a total human being and instead considering it a body containing a sick organ which is in need of care is a medical anathema.

It is within the discussions that are held between parents, families, and physicians immediately after birth that intense, emotional dilemmas arise. The disppointment and heartache-laden discussions about the newborn's potential (or lack thereof) must be open. Parents must be given the time to express their anquish. The physician's sensitivity and gentle counsel is rarely more crucial.

If we do not consider the whole patient, all variables, we fall into a situation where treatment could be given even if there is no gain or benefit to the newborn, in fact, there could be harm to the newborn. Father Richard McCormack supports the need to consider all variables. He stresses the fact that we must face the quality-of-life issue and that the most important criterion, as he sees it, is whether there is any "potential for human relationships."[9]

Much has been written regarding the relative value between early embryos, later fetuses, newborns, later infants, and the concept of personhood.[10] The claim of "personhood" and the right of a person to be treated is a commonly used argument to condemn the nontreatment of defective newborns. As Ramsey uses the argument of personhood in the attempts to force treatment even though substituted judgment would deem it unwise and unwarranted, others deny personhood to the newborn to support their position to withhold treatment.

As discussed in the preceding chapter, what is remarkable is how those who adamantly state that the fetus or newborn is a person do not grant the newborn the dignity of participating in the decision-making process by the use of the reasonable substituted judgment doctrine. To claim personhood and to then ignore the rights of that person is not only irrational and inconsistent but extremely dangerous in principle, since it assumes that the young people would not want society to decide for them as reasonable, intelligent, mature adults. It therefore flouts the most precious right inherent in a free society—freedom to decide.

It is precisely this attribute of personhood that forces one to look at the incompetent person, regardless of age, for advice in decision making. It is the only consistent approach to the management of persons who have never, regardless of reason, expressed what their desires would be under any given set of circumstances.

Those who advocate the nontreatment of seriously ill newborns, as exemplified by Mary Anne Warren,[11] Peter Singer,[12] and Michael Tooley,[13] deny personhood to newborns for various reasons. Tooley suggests that personhood demands a desire to continue to exist. Those who have the desire are persons, those who do not, and have never had the desire, are not persons. These proponents believe that the potential aspect of a being is simply not adequate for it to acquire the status of personhood. They demand some degree of relational awareness or consciousness. Although Tooley does not consider the newborn a person, he does appreciate the fact that if one concedes personhood to the newborn, termination of life may be warranted because the infant may prefer "death to continued existence or will do as soon as it becomes capable of having such a desire."[14]

Relational lack of development at the newborn stage is an important factor in decision making, but I suggest that the denial of rights to the tragic newborn on this basis would be an arbitrary concept, a tactic to validate the nontreatment of ill newborns. If we are to remain consistent, it is better to grant equal rights to all human life, regardless of the stage of its development. We cannot assume that the incompetent fetus or newborn has fewer rights than the incompetent adult.

If we accept the newborn as a person, and if substituted judgment is a valid and necessary approach to decision making, then it becomes a question of whether society is willing to allow a hopelessly ill newborn to die while keeping it comfortable and free of discomfort.

It is no less difficult for the decision makers to transfer themselves into the mind of an adult in coma, an adult whose past history we have no knowledge of, in order to reach a decision as to what that individual would desire, than it is to imagine themselves having the mind of the defective newborn and to determine what decision the infant would make as an adult, aware of the conditions at the newborn state and aware of the present relative absence of relational awareness and bonding.

If we are to act in the best interest of the newborn, we must consider all aspects of the situation in order for consent to be truly informed and therefore valid. This includes at minimum the state of its present life, the quality of its future life, the likelihood that it would be wanted and cared for at home, or institutionalized, the present level of its awareness, and the effect of its continued living upon parents and siblings. The newborn must be assumed to be as concerned with the life and welfare of his or her family as you or I are with our own families. To respect autonomy does not suggest any less respect of nonmaleficence or beneficence. But to preserve a tragically endowed newborn who would not survive without medical assistance and who would not, through substituted judgment, wish to survive is not only a misuse of technology but reflects disrespect of the dignity of personhood.

The process necessary to determine the newborn's best interest via reasonable substituted judgment may be difficult, agonizing, and heart-rending, but it is an effort that must be made for it is in the best interest of the newborn. To avoid making a decision is to make a decision, and to make a decision on limited data is to make an improper one.

Who should be burdened with the awesome task of evaluating the situation and reaching a decision that is reasonable and in the best interest of the newborn? The decision-making process must include a protective mechanism. The primary input should be made by the parents of the newborn. Their emotional distress is not such that reasonable judgments cannot be made, nor can their responsibility be denied or avoided. This is balanced by the physician, who must clarify all nuances of the problem from the medical point of view and discuss, not only as a physician but as a friend, the social factors as well. The parents must then decide what they believe would be in the best interests of the child. If their decision could result in the death of a newborn and if the physician believes this would be the decision he would make for his own newborn or the newborn of his daughter, then he must abide by the parents' decision not to treat. This approach is quite contrary to Weir, who believes that, "It is necessary to move beyond the ad hoc, whatever-the-physician-or-parents-think-best approach that currently characterizes selective nontreatment decisions."[15] Weir's attitude does not reflect the understanding that physicians are constantly involved in life-and-death decisions, that their approach is to do what is best for the patient within the constraints of the patient's wishes. Medical decisions are patient oriented, not society- or family oriented. The physician's dedication and loyalty is to the patient. The direction of the medical community is to treat and to preserve life, not to withhold treatment. The physician's psychological and traditional thrust toward continuing therapy, regardless of expense and subsequent effect upon society or the family, is a very strong protective mechanism that would nullify foolish decisions made by parents for a seriously ill newborn. Although this is not a perfect solution, it is a most reasonable one.

Courts have recognized family members as the most reasonable surrogate decision makers. The President's Commission resisted the claim that a legal guardian be appointed to make decisions for the incompetent person on the basis that "the cumbersomeness and costs of legal guardianship strongly militate against its use."[16] If the physician believes that the parental decision would result in an unwarranted death, the doctor is obligated to seek court assistance to negate what he or she believes is a wrong decision. If such a conflict arises, the courts must decide what would be reasonable substituted judgment for the newborn.

An alternative approach when there is doubt, or if there is a conflict between the parents and their physician, is to submit the problem to the hospital ethics committee for advice. If the ethics committee agrees with the parents that nontreatment would be the proper reasonable substituted judgment and the physician still is not convinced, then the doctor may seek court assistance. The court's judgment must be considered final.

The frame of reference to be used for substituted judgment is what the newborn would wish if it were aware of the present state of abnormality, the absence of any significant human quality relationships, the tragic physical, intellectual, psychological, and sociological aspects of the illness, and the effect of its life upon its parents. If a legal decision is required, the court must ask what the average person would wish to have done if that person had been so endowed at birth.

I believe that many, if not most, reasonable adults would, if they were able to, write a directive to their physicians that all supportive care to preserve life should cease at the newborn or early infancy stage if it were known that their minds were irrevocably damaged, so that even near-normal intellectual activities would not be possible, or if physical disability were severe, as in the case of paraplegia. This is supported by Dr. Arno Motulsky, who believes that, "Most parents in our society, if given the choice, would prefer an abortion of an affected fetus to a sick child who requires any but the most trivial treatment." [17]

I do not doubt that there is an element of fear of burden, unwarranted shame or guilt, ego, pride, and self-centered thoughts conjoined with such parental anguish. This must be part of the physician's awareness during the decision-making process. But in spite of these elements, traditionally, physicians and parents have been much more conservative and have not withheld medical treatment because of "trivial" problems. In actuality the trivial concept is never extrapolated to the newborn, while seriously defective newborns have been allowed to die. There is obviously no sharp line separating the tragic from the trivial. Pediatric neurosurgeon Donald Matson stated the following twenty-two years ago:

> In our clinic it is not customary to operate on newborn infants or those in the first few months of life with thoraco-lumbar or upper lumbar myelomeningoceles or myeloschises who exhibit complete sphincter paralysis and total paralysis below the upper lumbar segments. This is true whether or not there is significant hydrocephalus at the time.[18]

Complete paralysis below the waist with no control of bladder or bowels is a serious condition, not a trivial one.

In 1973, Raymond Duff and A. H. Campbell published their policy of nontreatment of the newborn and infants in the Yale–New Haven Hospital. During a period of thirteen months, forty-three newborn and early infants were allowed to die. The decision to withhold or discontinue therapy was made after frank discussion with parents. "When maximum treatment was viewed as unacceptable by families and physicians in our unit, there was a growing tendency to seek early death." Doctors Duff and Campbell expressed their anguish over "the awesome finality" and the "potential for error" but also realized that the problem must be faced. They believe that many physicians have not been totally candid regarding this issue:

> Physicians on the whole are reluctant to deal with [this] . . . there was a feeling that to "give up" was disloyal to the . . . profession.
>
> Since major research, teaching and patient-care efforts were being made, professionals were expected to discover, transmit and apply knowledge and skill; patients and families were supposed to cooperate fully [even] if they were not always grateful. Some physicians recognized that the wishes of families went against their own, but they were resolute. They (the doctors) commonly agreed that if they were the parents of very defective children, withholding treatment would be most desirable for them. However, they argued that aggressive treatment should be done for the children of others.[19]

This type of hypocrisy is not uncommon among physicians. Those who insist upon aggressively treating a patient when they would not recommend the same treatment for their own child, especially when parents are opposed to treatment, are contemptibly unethical. The only reasons for such actions are financial gain from performing surgery or unwarranted fear of criticism for not performing surgery. The lack of consent for surgery from parents should obviate that fear.

We must cease to assume that death is the ultimate harm to befall a patient. It may be in the best interest of a patient to leave life. The problem is to determine the parameters that exist on each side of the balancing scale. There is validity in the following statement by Dr. Gordon Avery.

> We sometimes unnecessarily prolong the misery of both baby and family when a hopeless situation could be terminated by withdrawing extraordinary therapy. We operate, ill-advisedly at times, on babies whose prognoses for meaningful life is nil. In my opinion, we would serve our patients better if we stopped to consider the consequences more carefully before using our new techniques.[20]

Most pediatricians would agree that newborns with certain disorders should not be treated. The problem among this group of physicians is not the moral issue but the parameters that determine which newborn should and which should not be treated.

It is time for the society of neonatologists and pediatricians to set forth general standards of development that warrant recommending to the parents medical or surgical treatment. Newborns who do not fulfill those criteria should only be kept completely free of discomfort.

A factor that unfortunately has to be considered in the management of a severely damaged newborn is the financial burden: "$100,000 is not an unusual hospital bill for the care of a tiny premature newborn."[21] Tremendous resources have to be made available for lifelong care in institutions, resources that can be used for the health of others. In this regard, the imposition of harm upon society in the form of a forced financial obligation must be seriously considered. The issue of triage and limitation of public funds for certain illnesses or defects will be discussed in chapter 10.

If a form is to be devised to expedite the withholding of medical and surgical treatment after a decision to do so has been made, it must at least include the following concepts.

> We, _____ , parents of baby _____ , do not give consent for any medical or surgical treatment to prolong the life of our newborn infant except for medication to prevent discomfort.

This burden, placed upon parents during the time of grief, must be accepted as a necessary act of responsibility. If parents cannot, because of emotional or religious reasons, make a decision whether to treat or not to treat, and if their doctor is willing to accept the responsibility to make the decision, the parents must at least make it safe for their doctor to do so. An approach that accomplishes this end and shares the burden with the physician, while easing the psychological weight on the parents, is to write a letter of authorization as follows:

> We, as parents of baby _____ , request and authorize our physician to manage the medical treatment of our newborn according to his best judgment, including the withholding of medical and surgical treatment with full understanding that death may ensue.

What else can parents do to prevent the treatment of their newborn without their consent? They must appreciate that they, not the doctor, are in the position of authority. If the physician demands to treat, when in the judgment of the parents treatment is ill-advised, they should add the following statement to the refusal-of-consent document. "If treatment is done without our written consent, we shall institute legal action for malpractice and assault and battery against the physicians in charge and the hospital facility."

NOTES

1. Gordon Avery, *Neonatology* (Philadelphia: J. B. Lippincott Co., 1987), p. 9.

2. John D. Arras, "The Effect of New Pediatric Capabilities and the Problem of Uncertainty," *The Hastings Center Report* 17 no. 6 (December 1987): 11.

3. Paul Ramsey, "Feticide/Infanticide Upon Request," *Religion in Life* 39 (1970): 170–86. p. 181.

4. Bernard Bart and Joseph Flether, "The Right to Die," *Atlantic Monthly* (April 1968): 63.

5. Ibid.

6. Paul Ramsey, *Ethics at the Edges of Life* (New Haven, Conn.: Yale University Press, 1978), p. 192.

7. Ibid., p. 215.

8. Robert Weir, *Selective Nontreatment of Handicapped Newborns* (New York: Oxford University Press, 1984), pp. 207-208.

9. Richard McCormack, "To Save or Let Die," *Journal of the American Medical Association* 229, no. 2 (July 8, 1974): 171-72.

10. Weir, *Selective Nontreatment of Handicapped Newborns*, pp. 190-94.

11. Mary Anne Warren, "On Infanticide," in *Today's Moral Problems*, R. Wasserstrom, ed. (New York: Macmillan Publishing Co., 1975), pp. 120-36.

12. Peter Singer, *Practical Ethics* (New York: Cambridge University Press, 1979).

13. Michael Tooley, "Decisions to Terminate Life and the Concept of Person," in *Ethical Issues Relating to Life and Death*, John Ladd, ed. (New York: Oxford University Press, 1979), p. 91.

14. Ibid, pp. 80-81.

15. Weir, *Selective Nontreatment of Handicapped Newborns*, p. 188.

16. President's Commission for the Study of Ethical Problems in Medicine and Biomedical and Behavioral Research, *Deciding to Forego Medical Therapy* (1983), p. 131.

17. Arno G. Motulsky et al., "Public Health and Long-Term Genetic Implications of Intrauterine Diagnosis and Selective Abortion," *Birth Defects* 7 (1971): 31.

18. Donald Matson, "Surgical Treatment of Myelomeningocele," *Pediatrics* 42, no. 2 (August 1968): 226.

19. Raymond S. Duff and A. H. M. Campbell, "Moral and Ethical Dilemmas in the Special Care Nursery," *The New England Journal of Medicine* 89 (October 25, 1973): 890–94.

20. Gordon Avery, quoted in Weir, p. 200.

21. Avery, *Neonatology,* p. 10.

8

Euthanasia

Euthanasia refers to the benevolent induction of an easy death. It is derived from the Greek words *eu* and *thanatos,* meaning "good" or "easy" death. The *Oxford English Dictionary* defines euthanasia as "the action of inducing a quiet or easy death."[1] The *American Heritage Dictionary* defines it as "the action of inducing the painless death of a person for reasons assumed to be merciful."[2] In 1869, William Lecky considered euthanasia an act of inducing easy death with the implication that the act would interfere with the process of life and thereby cause death.[3] This clear concept of euthanasia has become blurred in recent years.

The meaning of euthanasia has been broadened to include any action or lack of action that results in death regardless of whether or not it does so by interfering with the natural biological process (such as injecting an overdose of morphine) or by allowing nature to run its course (by removing life support systems). This expansion is unfortunate since it combines separate issues that complicate both ethical and legal problems. The concept of euthanasia arouses significant emotional reactions that tend to prevent dispassionate discussion; to broaden its meaning and then to attempt to clarify the meaning by applying modifiers such as *active* and *passive* only adds confusion to our reasoning.

The word *euthanasia* should remain restricted to those actions that cause death by interfering with the natural biological process. This is unlike the withholding of treatment, an act of *omission,* or the removal of life support systems, an act of *commission.* Both maneuvers may produce death but they do so by allowing the natural biological process to proceed to death. To limit euthanasia to acts that cause death by interfering with the natural course of life is consistent with the general public's sense of the word as being synonymous with mercy killing.

Although abortion is a subcategory of euthanasia since abortion deliberately interferes with the natural biological process, the traditional use of the words *euthanasia* and *infanticide* have been applied only to post-birth situations.

Freedom (the right of free choice), nonmaleficence, and beneficence are the prime factors that need to be evaluated when discussing euthanasia. Some writers, such as Gerard Hughes,[4] who eloquently expresses the Catholic point of view, make a strong argument suggesting that there is no moral difference between allowing someone to die and causing death by interfering with the biological process, since the end results are the same. This is not completely true. It does not take into consideration an important aspect of the doctor-patient relationship. The physician is a guardian of the patient. If the patient consciously (or through a prior directive, or reasonable substituted judgment) refuses further medical care or demands cancellation of existing medical care, the wishes must be respected except under very unusual circumstances, regardless of the physician's philosophy or desires, since treatment without consent is not acceptable. To do so would violate the rules of morality, as well as the law. But the patient does not have the right to impose upon the physician or any other person an obligation to kill. Euthanasia not only involves the right of an individual to die, but the burden upon someone else to interfere with nature to cause death. This is contrary to the physician's usual role unless it is assumed that to induce death under certain circumstances may be considered reasonable therapy. This problem concerning the physician's role is also exposed by the humane concept expressed by H. Tristram Englehardt: "If life is not always better than death, it may be beneficent to expedite death rather than 'let nature take its course.' "[5] This, however, suggests that benevolence would not only sanction euthanasia, even as I define it, but may obligate the physician to perform it. But now we encounter the problem of the obligation of the physician to act in a beneficent manner when the emotional cost to him or her may be too high.

As discussed in chapter 1, there is a moral obligation to do good as long as the act of beneficence is not too demanding or harmful to the person in a position to do good. Although this moral obligation may sanction an act of euthanasia, it does not obligate a physician to comply with someone's desire to die if such an act is personally repugnant. The physician is the agent of the patient only to the extent that he or she is not forced to act contrary to personal judgment.

It is common practice for physicians to refrain from treating or to remove life support systems, both of which result in death. But not all physicians would be willing to inject an overdose of medication to cause death. To perform euthanasia must therefore be balanced against the physician's wishes to comply. The emotional burden that accompanies interfering with the biological process is enough to separate euthanasia from the question of stopping or withholding medical treatment, even if the legal ramifications are the same.

Since ancient times, many have believed that mercy killing is morally justified if it ends the suffering of a dying patient and if that patient requests it. But at the same time it has been vehemently condemned by others. Two arguments against the legalization of euthanasia are, first, the possibility that families, burdened by the existence of a chronically ill parent, may encourage them to die, and second, that the sanctioning of euthanasia, regardless of how well controlled it may be, may result in a general callousness toward the elderly or chronically ill person. In essence, condemnation of euthanasia, aside from religious doctrines, is primarily based upon the fear that legalization of mercy killing would devalue human life and lead to attitudes that would permit the destruction of those not requesting death. This fear, although understandable, is probably not warranted. In spite of the rampant destruction and death throughout the world there has not been a significant change in our attitudes toward death. Societies have not become more callous. In fact, most states have abolished capital punishment. The fear that legalization of euthanasia would serve as a wedge does not bear up under scrutiny. Euthanasia is not a crime in Switzerland, Norway, Germany, and Peru. It is legally a criminal offense in the Netherlands but the courts have accepted the practice under extenuating circumstances. Societal attitudes toward death are no more callous in these societies than in our own. Misuse has not been shown to exist in those nations that have approved it. Englehardt agrees: the fear that social acceptance of euthanasia would destroy our ethical sense is not warranted.

> History shows, the moral fabric does not appear to depend on condemning infanticide. The fabric seems quite able to sustain a highly advanced and intricate culture with notions of generosity and magnanimity, while not condemning the killing of newborns in general, or deformed neonates in particular.[6]

Regardless of historical patterns and of the many cultures that approve of euthanasia, and in spite of nature's tendency to eliminate the seriously deformed, we cannot assume that such indicators validate euthanasia. As acknowledged by Helga Kuhse and Peter Singer[7] and supported by Earl Shelp[8] and Stephen Post,[9] one "cannot validly argue from the fact that something is widespread to the judgment that it is good."[10] Yet, we must be skeptical of Post's remark that, "There seems no reason to undermine one of its obvious strengths, a conviction that newborns are not simply parental property, but rather a part of the moral community."[11]

This idea may lead us back to ancient Greece, where the individual was the property of the state. This is anathema to anyone who holds individual freedom precious.

There are ethicists, exemplified by Arthur Dyck,[12] who argue against euthanasia by stating that,

> "It is merciful not to kill" and that "Any act . . . of taking a human life is wrong" unless for example, "a person's effort to prevent someone's death may lead to the death of the attacker." This can be justified since "it is an act of saving a life. . . . If it were simply an act of taking a life, it would be wrong."[12]

But in Dyck's general discussion it is apparent that his position is primarily based upon fear of wrongful extrapolation of the use of euthanasia. Dyck agrees that mercy and kindness are moral obligations, and that the deliberate shortening of a human life dying in anguish would be as merciful as ending the anguish of a dying deer. But he also believes that killing with the intent to relieve suffering is wrong. The problem is not whether such an act would be merciful or justified; the danger lies in establishing doctrines or principles that can be misused. Dyck is not alone in believing that to kill out of kindness for the relief of suffering can be extrapolated to the point of absurdity.

Before discussing if euthanasia should be legalized, when would it ever be applicable? There are five situations in which euthanasia might be considered. The first situation involves the patient who is competent and who can at least partially feed him or herself. That patient has the ability to commit suicide. Euthanasia in such circumstances would be inadvisable for two reasons. First, the patient is not given a good psychological opportunity to change his or her mind during the last second. It is easier for a patient to reconsider options if contemplating suicide in total privacy. The fact that a decision has been made, discussed, evaluated, and navigated through the necessary precautionary logistics that would involve the taking of life places the patient in a committed position which, especially in the presence of others, would make it difficult to retract the request for death. Second, if the patient can gracefully commit suicide with assistance, why should a burden be placed upon someone in society to end life? Under these circumstances, if suicide appears to be warranted, a law to allow assisted suicide would be the proper solution, not euthanasia.

The second situation involves the mentally competent patient who is physically incapable of committing suicide. This would be extremely rare. The Zygmaniak case is an example. In 1973, Lester Zygmaniak shot his brother, who had become quadriplegic following an accident, after his brother adamantly begged Lester to end his life.[13] This was an act of love filled with extreme anguish. Lester's motivation was admirable, but his act was probably unwise since it was performed too soon after his brother's accident. He did not realize that with time and proper psychological help his brother could possibly adapt to his tragic condition. If the demand to die were made after all help had failed, then we would be faced with a problem that can only be solved by euthanasia or self-starvation, unless we wish to force the person to live in a state of mental if not physical anguish.

The third situation involves the adult who is in irreversible coma or in a permanent, noncognitive state, such as Karen Ann Quinlan or Nancy Beth Cruzan, whose parents had requested that their daughters be allowed to die. In such cases either a directive is provided to the physician, a durable power of attorney is written while the patient is competent, or the request to die is based upon the patient's previously expressed desires to the family or the physician. Under these circumstances, the prolongation of life by treating complications of the illness or by providing food and water through tubes is certainly not warranted. Any effort to prolong life would be against the wishes and consent of the patient and therefore wrongful since there would be no extenuating factors that would warrant treatment without consent. If this is true, would it not be merciful, especially if requested by the patient in a prior directive, to perform euthanasia? I believe so, but it would probably not be necessary if artificial means of hydrating and feeding such patients ceased, and the patient were merely kept comfortable. Under such circumstances death would ensue within a few days.

A fourth category is the mentally retarded or severely physically handicapped newborn. Infanticide is euthanasia at the newborn stage. Infanticide is an ancient practice that was widely accepted by both illiterate and more advanced, literate societies.[14-15] The motivation underlying such actions included elimination of deformities that would prevent self-sustenance and that were associated with ominous superstitious signs, e.g., economic factors and simple population control.[16] It was common in the Pacific islands, China, Africa, South America, as well as early Greece and Rome. Both Plato and Aristotle were firm advocates of infanticide.[17] It was common in Europe until the nineteenth century. The major impetus against infanticide has been the Judaic and Christian abhorrence of the act. It was this theological thrust that molded Western attitudes.

Some hold that its (the Christian church's) opposition rested primarily upon concepts such as those of stewardship, of man's sociospiritual solidarity, of life as a gift from God, and of man as God's creation. Other writers, including historians of ethics such as Westermarck and Lecky, maintain that the main source of the opposition to infanticide was the belief that man was immortal, together with the belief that unbaptized infants would endure eternal torment in hell.[18]

If we consider the newborn a nonperson as suggested by Englehardt, then the arguments against infanticide become insignificant, for a nonperson can reasonably be considered as only a living organism, not endowed with humanhood, and with which parents may or may not have an emotional tie. Although this may be disturbing emotionally, it would, as Englehardt suggests, be "difficult to mount a plausible, nonculturally biased, strong argument against infanticide. The best that can be produced is a speculative, circumstantial argument."[19] Under these circumstances the autonomy and privacy of the parents should theoretically prevail. The basis for decision making may include the elements of anguish for the future of the newborn, parental anguish, the potential burden on society, and economic factors.

I believe it is imperative to remain consistent in the application of ethical principles. If, as discussed in the chapter on abortion, we consider any stage of the developing or aging human as a person regardless of condition, and therefore the conceptus is considered a person, reasonable substituted judgment that would be applied to decisions affecting the conceptus or fetus should be equally applicable to the newborn. If a decision is made to withhold therapy on the basis of reasonable substituted judgment for a tragic newborn, to allow death to slowly take place appears relatively inhumane. It then becomes reasonable to utilize euthanasia. To prolong suffering is to permit harm. By not resorting to euthanasia we are not acting in a beneficent manner and therefore we are not acting ethically. Weir suggests that if, after careful scrutiny, life-prolonging treatment is no longer considered to be in the best interests of the child and the decision has already been made to allow the newborn to die, and it is quite clear that the child is not going to die quickly but is going to endure prolonged suffering in the absence of treatment, a decision should be made to end the child's life quickly and painlessly.[20] A tragic situation arose with the birth of a newborn with Down's syndrome and duodenal atresia (a blockage of the small intestine which can be corrected surgically).[21] The decision was to allow the newborn to die. In the mother's words, "It would be unfair to the other children of the household to raise them with a mongoloid." The parents were informed that the degree of mental retardation could not be predicted. The newborn was put in a side room and after eleven days it died. Regardless of whether we agree or disagree with the decision, a more humane approach would have been euthansia.

In regard to acts of infanticide, Ramsey, who so adamantly opposes abortion and infanticide, inserts the thought that is totally independent of the use of substituted judgment and suggests that direct killing may be warranted as an exception to what he terms a generally justifiable practice. In his discussion of the management of the Lesch-Nyhan child, he states that, "The moral reason for continuing to distinguish between allowing to die and direct killing loses its force when the patient becomes totally inaccessible."[22]

The fifth category includes the mentally retarded older child or adult, who through reasonable substituted judgment would request not to be kept alive. There are two subgroups in this category: those who are so badly brain damaged that they are and will be permanently unaware of relationships, and those who are aware of relationships. It is at this point that we approach the fear expressed by Ramsey.[23]

Ramsey believed that the principles used to validate abortion may be used to validate the nontreatment of seriously defective newborns, and then possibly become extrapolated to permit unwarranted killing of defective older children. This fear of unwarranted extrapolation becomes very poignant at later stages of life because the defective newborns may have developed, depending upon the degree of damage, some form of personality, some bonding with parents or guardians, some awareness of life with obvious sensibilities.

Those patients in the first subgroup, essentially permanently unaware of relationships, are in the same position as the fourth category involving tragic newborns for which euthanasia becomes a viable option. This includes older children or adults who are in need of medical care to preserve life and are so severely mentally deficient that they seem not to have any sense of the difference between living and dying. This includes cases such as the Tay-Sachs or Lesch-Nyhan child, as well as the severely mentally retarded person unaware of his own uninhibited defecation and urination, lying in a corner detached from the world, and the hopelessly global aphasic patient who can neither comprehend nor respond to language. These heartbreaking groups, if ever they had the opportunity to write a directive to their physicians, would in all probability state that they would not wish to live in their present states. If this be so, prolongation of life would not be warranted. At maximum, medical care would be warranted to maintain comfort, but not to prolong life. Artificial life-support systems would not be acceptable. It is for this group that euthanasia could seriously be considered with good rationale.

The second subgroup, those who are incompetent but aware of relationships, must never be considered as candidates for euthanasia. The potential for misuse is too great. When a decision is made to let life end at the newborn stage, it is at a time when the newborn's sense of awareness is minimal and the newborn-parent relational component is essentially absent. In this respect, the newborn is quite different from that of an older child. The Down's syndrome patient at birth is not the same as at the age of ten. It is obvious that a happy, gentle, and loving child afflicted with Down's syndrome would not see death as an alternative to his or her handicapped life.

It is only by establishing the above safeguard that Ramsey's legitimate fear of misuse or wrongful extrapolation of the abortion principle can be alleviated.

The Netherlands supreme court sanctioned euthanasia if the following conditions were satisfied: (1) the patient's condition was intolerable, with no hope of improvement; (2) relief was not possible; (3) the patient was competent; (4) the request originated with the patient and the patient was persistent; (5) consultation was obtained and both physicians agreed with the reasonableness of the request.[24] U.S. criminal law holds that euthanasia, which is a willful act, is, regardless of motivation, and regardless of consent, an act of first degree murder.[25-27] Even the assistance of suicide is considered a criminal act in many states. But in spite of legal statutes, and although motivation is not a legally acceptable defense,[28] the attitude of our courts has been more reasonable. Altruistic motivation has been considered an extenuating factor in judging homicides. This gap between the written law and actual practice as it pertains to mercy killing is an embarrassment to law. We should modify our law as other countries have done and accept motivation as a legitimate defense in court, especially since we already do so in practice. We should not have to resort to legal subterfuge such as temporary insanity pleas. The fact that our law is not consistent with our actions is, as expressed by Dr. Eliot Slater, "a patent absurdity."[29]

SUGGESTIONS FOR CHANGE

Although I believe that euthanasia is morally correct under certain circumstances, I also believe that any act of euthanasia, as here defined, should be subject to review by an ethics committee or ombudsman because of the danger of wrongful extrapolation. This should be done prior to the act. If the act has been done and if circumstances are suspect, a legal charge should be instituted. As Annas suggests, we must feel the pressure of responsibility of euthanasia in regard to the tragic newborn.[30]

In order to expedite this change, two suggestions are made. First, homicide law should be amended to allow motivation, intent, and consent, actual or implied, to be an integral part of the homicide defense. Second, we should allow a judge, arbitrator, regional ombudsman, or ethics committee to evaluate the case and to give or deny consent. The decision would be based upon whether the motive underlying an act of euthanasia is that of kindness and respect toward the patient, a desire to help the patient, and an act consistent with reasonable substituted judgment or with the expressed written or implied desires of the patient. If motivation is other than benevolence toward the patient then the act becomes suspect as being some other form of homicide.

The crucial factor underlying the acceptance of euthanasia is the motivation to be merciful and the safeguard of consent whenever possible. Because of these two factors, euthanasia can never be equated with other forms of homicide, or with the acts of brutality as performed by the Nazis.

Recently, recommendations have been proposed in California and Washington for legislative action to approve euthanasia.[31] Both proposals failed to become law. They combined the issues of euthanasia, as I define it, with doctor-assisted suicide and the right to refuse medical therapy. I am skeptical of efforts to legalize euthanasia. There are too many adverse ramifications. The proposals, as stated by A. R. Demac, "provide a sledge-hammer where a feather is needed."[32] A better alternative would be the suggested modification of homicide law to include motivation factors as a legitimate defense. Since homicide is acceptable in cases of self-defense, it may be considered acceptable if the motive is mercy. Obviously, parameters would have to be set that would include request and approval by the patient, or by the family if the patient is incompetent, combined with consultation and perhaps approval by the hospital director or ethics committee.

NOTES

1. *Oxford English Dictionary* (New York: Oxford University Press, 1971).

2. *American Heritage Dictionary* (Boston: Houghton Mifflin Co., 1979).

3. William B. Lecky, *History of European Morals from Augustus to Charlemagne* (1869).

4. Gerard J. Hughes, "Killing and Let Die," *The Month* 226, no. 1290 (1975): 42–45.

5. H. T. Englehardt, *The Foundation of Bioethics* (New York: Oxford University Press, 1986): p. 316.

6. Ibid., p. 229.

7. Helga Kuhse and Peter Singer, *Should the Baby Live* (New York: Oxford University Press, 1985), p. 108.

8. Earl Shelp, *Born to Die? Deciding the Fate of Critically Ill Newborns* (New York: Free Press, 1986), p. 154.

9. Stephen Post, "History, Infanticide and Imperiled Newborns," *Hastings Center Report* 18, no. 4 (August-September 1988): 14–17.

10. Kuhse and Singer, *Should the Baby Live,* p. 108.

11. Stephen Post, "History, Infanticide and Imperiled Newborns," p. 15.

12. Arthur Dyck, "Beneficent Euthanasia and Benemortasia," in *Beneficent Euthanasia,* Marvin Kohl, ed. (Buffalo, N.Y.: Prometheus Books, 1975), p. 124.

13. Paige Mitchell, *Act of Love: The Killing of George Zygmaniak* (New York: Knopf Publishing Co., 1976).

14. Englehardt, *The Foundation of Bioethics,* p. 228.

15. Edward Westermarck, *Origin and Development of the Moral Ideas* (London: Macmillan Publishers, 1924), pp. 394–413.

16. *Encyclopaedia Britannica* Vol. 12 (Chicago: William Benton Publishers, 1958), p. 323.

17. Michael Tooley, "Infanticide: A Philosophical Perspective" in *Encyclopedia of Bioethics* (New York: The Free Press, 1978), p. 742.

18. Ibid., p. 743.

19. Englehardt, *The Foundation of Bioethics*, p. 229.

20. Robert Weir, *Selective Nontreatment of Handicapped Newborns* (New York: Oxford University Press, 1984), p. 221.

21. James M. Gustafson, "Mongolism, Parental Desires, and the Right to Life," *Perspectives in Biology and Medicine* 16, no. 4 (Summer 1973): 529-57.

22. Paul Ramsey, *Ethics at the Edges of Life* (New Haven, Conn.: Yale University Press, 1978), p. 216.

23. Paul Ramsey, "Feticide/Infanticide Upon Request," *Religion in Life* 39 (1970): 170-86, p. 181.

24. P. V. Admiraal, *Justifiable Euthanasia: A Manual for the Medical Profession* (Amsterdam, The Netherlands: Vervoor Vrijwillige Euthanasie, 1980).

25. *Martin* v. *Commonwealth* (1946) 184Va 1009, 1018, 1019, 37se/2d 43, 47.

26. *People* v. *Conley* (1966) 64 CAL. 2d 310, 322, 49 CAL Rptr. 815.

27. *People* v. *Dessauer* (1952) 38 CAL. 2d 547, 241, PAC. 2ed 238.

28. Motivation is recognized in homicide in Belgium, France, Germany, The Netherlands, Switzerland, Uruquay, Peru, Iran, Czechoslovakia, and Sweden.

29. Eliot Slater, quoted in O. Ruth Russell, "Moral and Legal Aspects of Euthanasia," *The Humanist* (July-August 1974), p. 22.

30. George Annas, personal communication, 1990.

31. (a) Humane and Dignified Death Initiative. California State Legislative Proposal #7185. Sponsored by Americans against Human Suffering, Glendale, California; (b) State of Washington Initiative 119.

32. A. R. Demac, "Thoughts on Physician-Assisted Suicide," *Western Journal of Medicine* 148 (February 1988): 229.

9

Human Experimentation

There are many categories and gradations of human experimentation. They range from noninvasive studies such as demographic analyses of ethnic groups in poverty areas to the experimental transplantation of heart and lungs into a dying patient. Regardless of the category or the quality of the study, the principles involved are the same.

Since the emphasis of this work is medicine, my discussion is restricted to experiments that involve medical or surgical studies of the human body. The problems pertaining to sociological or nonhuman biological experiments will not be discussed. All four ethical principles become pertinent in human experimentation programs.

The purpose of research is to advance human knowledge in the hope that it may benefit society for the common good. But in spite of the fantastic advances in both knowledge and technical sophistication, it is not quite certain that people are better or happier as a result of research studies, although we may live longer.

We have been inclined to surround research with a mantle of sanctity. To challenge experimentation is to challenge progress, but what makes human beings unique is not su-

173

perior reasoning, nor sophistication and technical prowess, but the ability to understand and feel the needs of fellow human beings—to feel compassion and tenderness, and to respect the dignity of others. The value of knowledge gained through experimentation is never so great that we may neglect our respect for one another.

All too often, both society and the scientist may be so blind in the thirst for knowledge and the status associated with it that the rights and safety of individuals are ignored. Although the expansion of knowledge should not be deprecated, its relationship to moral values must be reexamined. If individual rights are ignored in the pursuit of knowledge, it may be more dangerous and destructive than the inhibition of scientific progress. In the words of Hans Jonas, failure to safeguard human rights may lead to "the erosion of those moral values whose loss, possibly caused by too ruthless a pursuit of scientific progress, would make its most dazzling triumphs not worth having."[1]

A healthy scientific dedication and respect for moral values are not mutually exclusive. But a conflict of interest exists and the researcher must face it. There is a psychological and practical need for the scientist to do research, especially in an academic environment. This need may cloud the researcher's sense of ethics. The pressures to publish or perish are real.

Human experimentation is part of everyday medicine and surgery. All diagnostic and therapeutic procedures demand that the physician balance the danger of performing or not performing a diagnostic study or treatment against its potential benefit to the patient. Within every modality that the physician uses or does not use, uncertainty as to the result is a given. The element of doubt and danger is always present. People react differently to any given program. Because of this variable, all forms of therapy and diagnostic tests, from taking one's temperature to removing a brain tumor, are part of an ongoing human experimentation program through the accumulation of necessary data. The statistical significance of any treatment or test must be determined. The true relationship of an approach to a disease process can only be determined by long-term, continuous observation. It is only through continuous evaluation of new as well as commonplace drugs that we slowly determine efficacy, variation in dosage factors, and the common or uncommon side effects of these medications. Even the daily use of aspirin is still part of a human experimentation program that has been going on for decades. We still do not know all there is to know about aspirin. Every operation is to some extent part of a human experiment. The experimental aspect of the surgical procedure may at times be more significant than simply enlarging a database. It has been a standard practice for me as a neurosurgeon to modify my surgical technique regarding a brain or spinal lesion to see if a new angle of approach, a newly designed instrument, or a change in the timing of surgery may be of value to the patient. These slight new changes, or new instruments, are used without specific prior discussion with the patient. It is part of the everyday surgical amphitheater. This is not the type of human experimentation that demands an amplified consent. But one must be aware that there may be a fine line to be drawn as to when the new instrument to be used or the new approach warrants disclosure to the patient. This depends upon the significance of the variation. At the present time we are testing a new type of brain retractor support.* It is similar in principle to present devices. This new design is theoretically easier for the surgeon to control and safer for the patient. Since it is essentially a variation of existing designs, although it is new and therefore experimental, there does not appear to be any need to discuss it with the patient before

---

*A device that holds the brain in position when operating within its depths.

or after surgery. However, the experimental use of the eximer laser to ream out obstructed arteries to the heart was and is dangerous enough that detailed informed consent was necessary before it could be used. Patients had to understand the risks involved, especially that of burning a hole in the side of the artery, which could produce serious bleeding. The decision as to whether the degree of difference between the procedure, drug, or instrument that is to be tried is significantly different from what is commonly used, or in common practice, will vary with the integrity, the aggressiveness, and the attitude of the experimenter.

Since modern medical care is the direct result of human experimentation, all who receive medical care have gained from prior human testing. But this does not imply that those who have benefited owe a debt that demands participation in human experimentation. Prior experiments were not authorized or requested by those who now reap the benefits. Fundamentally, there is no ethical imperative directing any member of society to participate in a risky scientific experiment, but there is, as previously discussed in chapter 1, the concept that "people should do good." This carries with it a soft obligation to present and future society to participate or to support such efforts.

Scientists have the right to pursue knowledge and to experiment. But this does not include the right to experiment upon others without consent. To do so would be an invasion of privacy and an assault upon their person.

Although there is a strong sense of social consciousness and social responsibility among many scientists, society cannot but remember the brutally aggressive, immoral human experiments performed by German physicians during the Second World War. Society must always be on guard. The motivation, brilliance, and assumed integrity of the experimenter cannot be accepted as reason enough to not worry about the rights of the person upon whom the experiment is to be performed. We cannot move along simply on the basis of trust. We cannot depend upon P. W. Bridgman's perception that, "The scientist has a humility almost religious."[2]

After years of sitting on human experimentation committees, I am convinced that this comment by Dr. Bridgman is a glamorous and unwarranted view of the attitude of most scientists. Their humility is often lost in the enthusiasm of work and may only reflect a scientist's awe of science rather than respect for other people. All too often, those of talent fall prey to their enthusiasm and innovative thoughts. This may result in a cavalier approach to the patient and to society.

Researchers should have a sense of responsibility for the effect of their work, but that does not mean they must be held publicly accountable for the misuse or undesirable effects of the research. But the consequences of the use and possible misuse of new data should be taken into consideration. It is for this reason that there has been so much discussion regarding genetic engineering of bacteria and the development of new strains whose effect upon society may yet be unknown. If the new data can be dangerous or misused, then the research team must make every effort to prevent that misuse before it is published. This may not always be feasible. Responsibility toward the common good holds true for sociological as well as biological and physical studies. This sense of social responsibility is as important as the scholarship, integrity and meticulous attention to detail that scientists must have in their work.

The motivation of the subject of experiments falls into four main categories: the desire to be cured of disease, monetary gain, a sense of obligation to society, and pleasure from the sense of exploration associated with participation in an experiment. Probably many of us would accept experimentation upon ourselves if the experiment were properly designed, performed by qualified personnel, properly supervised, and if we were unfortunately in one of the following conditions:

1. suffering from a deadly or incapacitating disease, which is not treatable, in the hope that the experiment will produce a cure or prevent the progression of the disease;

2. engaged in studies or therapy in which additional studies of an experimental nature would be virtually risk-free in order to help others at little cost to ourselves; or

3. in a position of financial need.

Most of us would not accept experimentation upon ourselves while normal, if there were any discomfort or serious risk. But a slight risk would often be acceptable if we were convinced that the results of the experiment would be of potential value to others.

The relationship between the experimenter and the subject is in many respects dependent upon the circumstances and character of the experiment, but, regardless of the conditions, the single most crucial factor is that of consent. This consent must be much more detailed than the informed consent in the usual doctor-patient relationship. It is unwarranted to equate the degree of consent used for standard medical and surgical treatment with the consent needed for human experimentation. Standard consent demands that the most common and serious problems and alternatives be discussed with the patient. Consent for human experimentation demands that *all known data*, not just the most important details, must be explained to the participant. *All known risks and all known potential benefits must be disclosed.* The significance of unknown possibilities must be discussed with the subject. The participants must fully appreciate the fact that not all the risks are known and that there may be hidden dangers.

Any form of persuasion is not acceptable. This is unlike the ordinary patient-doctor relationship in which the physician is obligated to try to persuade the patient to do what is in his or her best interest.

Arrogance and callousness were dramatically revealed in the defense of a human experiment in which live cancer cells were injected into patients without their knowledge.[3] When the experiment was exposed, the defense argued as follows:

> Medical ethics do not require the full disclosure to a patient of all conceivable risks and all relevant information as the basis for obtaining patient(s) consent to a medical procedure. The amount of information imparted to a patient must bear some resemblance to the risk of some particular procedure. Where there is no substantial risk of harm to a patient, the information imparted to him may be kept at a minimum.[4]

In an experiment, who is to evaluate the word "substantial"? Is that not the patient's prerogative rather than the scientist's? It is of interest to know that in this situation the experimenter did not perform the experiment upon himself. He agreed with the philosophy that, "There are relatively few skilled cancer researchers, and it seems stupid to take even the little risk."[5]

This aggressive approach reflects the relative egocentricity, arrogance, and insensitivity of some scientists. The incident also reflects the unwarranted lofty status given to the importance of research. Even an experienced physician such as Dr. I. S. Ravdin fell prey to this worship of research. He supported the ethics of the live cancer cell experiment by stating,

> Research in the field of host response and immune reactions is likely to provide the first important breakthrough in the treatment of malignant diseases. It is men like Dr. Southam who are best prepared to accomplish this highly desirable breakthrough.[6]

No one denies the possible potential value of such research. One only questions the right of a scientist to fool and take advantage of another person.

The question of deception, so necessary in doubleblind* drug evaluation studies, must be faced. It is always difficult to assume a truly positive or negative stand. But at minimum the patient must be aware that the specific drug to be used or not used cannot be revealed. If the patient is aware of this factor, then it is no longer deception since it becomes acceptance of an unknown with consent.

In view of the possibility that some aspects are not fully understood by the patient, the experimenter is ethically bound under the factor of nonmaleficence not to accept consent at face value. To proceed without fully understood consent is to do harm. As a result, formally written consent does not nullify the experimenter's obligation to protect the subject.

The element of duress inherent within illness makes vulnerability and exploitation serious concerns for researchers. Elderly and timid people may agree to an experimental procedure because they cannot easily say no. The scientist must be sensitive to their vulnerability and not take advantage or exploit the situation. To do so would be unethical in spite of consent. All too often those who need care at publicly supported institutions may be foreigners with severe language barriers, elderly people who are forgetful and not fully aware, or people with little educational background. They are frequently not in a position to fully understand the ramifications of an experiment. Others may be simply poor as well

---

*An experimental study performed on a group of people with the same illness. Fifty percent will receive medication A and 50 percent will receive medication B. Neither the patients nor the doctors know which group receives which medication until the experiment has been completed and the clinical effect has been tabulated. Then one may, without bias, decide which drug was most effective in treating that specific illness.

as ill. Their need, their psychological state of fatigue, and the ambience within a hospital continue to place them in a position to be easily intimidated by an experimenter. There is a unique relationship between authority, the scientist's image, and the psychology of those who are ill. Their susceptibility to suggestion and to authority must be appreciated. Because such subjects are vulnerable and there may be complex motivations which lead them to accept a research program, the experimenter is obliged to protect the patient as well as the patient's family. This holds true regardless of the motivation of the person who is willing to undergo experimentation.

Experimental subjects must have the right to cancel their participation in an experiment. If to do so would ruin the experiment, the subject must be informed of this result, and must be made to realize that there is at least a prima facie obligation to continue. Nonetheless, if there is too much stress or undesirable reactions, the participant/experimentee must be free to stop in spite of the contractual agreement. Obviously if the contract is broken and remuneration was part of the agreement, this may have to be forfeited.

Society has every right to be concerned with all aspects of human experimentation under the principles of nonmaleficence and the common good. First and foremost, it must question whether individual rights are to be subordinated to society's desire for knowledge. Different political societies will answer this question differently. Our society, which believes that the individual does not exist for the welfare of others—in fact, the converse is the case—does not easily permit human experimentation without consent. An ethic that places society above individual freedom may feel justified in coercing its members to further the common good. As a result, our ethical values would appear to inhibit human experimentation and therefore the advance of science. But that same morality enhances the dignity of individuals and allows our research to be more critically evaluated without political constraints. As a result, our scientific progress has been excellent.

If we ever lose respect for the hierarchy that places individual rights above scientific goals, we will set a precedent that may lead to political and social disaster. We would be destroying the preciousness of autonomy and nonmaleficence, and in so doing dehumanize society. Such actions could easily spread from the scientific to the social arena, where individual freedom and privacy could be devalued.

It is quite apparent that the burden of experimentation falls upon those less fortunate than others, those who may have the most to gain from the experiment, namely, the sick and the poor, which includes most prisoners. The common denominator within this group is the element of duress. Duress is inherent within those who participate in human experiments except for those who participate with a high sense of moral purpose to help society. The Belmont Report of the National Commission for the Protection of Human Subjects of Biomedical and Behavioral Research discusses the general guidelines for protection of human subjects of research.[7]

EXPERIMENTING ON PRISONERS

This section, although focused only on prisoners, is somewhat extensive since the problems raised should help to clarify the ethical principles involved in all human experiments. The issues were well presented during the consideration of this problem by the national commission mentioned above. The conclusion of the commission, after much debate, severely limited experimentation on prisoners.

The arguments presented before the national commission by those who oppose prisoner experimentation include at least the following:

1. Adequate medical facility and personnel necessary to care for possible complications of experimentation are not readily available.

2. Experiments are frequently ineptly performed.

3. Experiments are frequently inadequately supervised.

4. Prisoners are not properly compensated for their participation.

5. Most of the research is nontherapeutic as far as the prisoner is concerned. In other words, the results of the research study would probably not be of any medical benefit to the prisoner.

6. Prisoners as a group bear a disproportionate share of the burdens of research or bear those burdens without receiving a commensurate share of the benefits that ultimately derive from research.[8]

7. Prisoners are not able to give truly free consent since they are constrained by their incarceration.

The first three arguments are certainly valid. Obviously the parameters surrounding research on prisoners should be no less rigid than those applied to research involving any other citizen. The inequities, the inept research, the research without consent, the unwarranted risky research, the bad research is no more pertinent to prisoners than any other individuals. If it is bad, it is bad across the board. If it is inept, it is inept throughout. One can list unwise, inept, and unethical research programs performed in prisons as well as outside of penal institutions. Proper control must apply to all. This holds true regardless of whether or not the subject is in or out of prison. If an experiment is not properly supervised, designed, and executed it should not be done anywhere. If peer control has been lax, then it should be corrected. If medical facilities are not adequate, the experimenter must cancel the program or build new facilities. Obviously, the responsibility to supply medical care needed during the experiment or as a result of the experiment, must be that of the experimenter. If as a result of the experiment the subject becomes disabled, there must be provisions for disability through insurance.

Equity, the fairness rule, demands that prisoners be paid comparably to free volunteers. If equity requirements are not fulfilled, then prisoner experimentation would be exploitation. This would constitute maleficence. To take advantage of their poverty to reduce the cost of the experiment is no less exploitation than an unfair and unethical exploitation of an ill patient at a county hospital.

The remuneration received must be commensurate with the risks and effort. Monies received for experimentation purposes should be directed to the person upon whom the experiment is being done rather than placed into a prisoner welfare fund for improvement of the prison system. The prisoner should have the right of full compensation. If it is his or her wish to apportion part of the funds to the prison welfare system, that is the prisoner's prerogative, but it should not be taken out of the fair fee. Any fees that are above what would be equitable and fair could then be given to the prison welfare fund.

It is clearly against the common good to purchase the consent of prisoners by offering them consideration at the time of parole. We have to assume that prisoners are not incarcerated simply to pay a debt, but rather to protect society from a dangerous person, to deter that person and others from committing crime, or to rehabilitate a criminal. If this is so, then participation in an experiment should not in any way alter their time in prison. If the time stipulated was deemed advisable to protect society, to rehabilitate, or to deter future crime, then that time must not be changed. There is much truth to the following statement by Edmond Cahn:

There is not much to say for a society that sends a burglar to prison for 10 years and gives him to understand that he can be free in five if he subjects himself to medical experiments.[9]

The question of whether or not the research is therapeutic to the prisoner is irrelevant. Most normal volunteers who are not prisoners do not benefit from research either. It is the monetary compensation that is of great benefit to the prisoner. The fact that prisoners bear a disproportionate share of the research is also irrelevant as long as a desire to do it is fully protected within the limits of the experiment and fully compensated. We must be aware that our attitude toward prisoners may be somewhat more callous than our attitude toward a cancer patient. This may lead to a tendency to exploit them.

The most important criticism of prisoner experimentation refers to the question of free consent. The national commission commented:

It seems at first glance that the principle of respect for persons requires that prisoners not be deprived the opportunity to volunteer for research. . . . When persons seem regularly to engage in activities which, were they stronger or in better circumstances, they would avoid, respect dictates that they be protected against those forces that appear to compel their choices. It has become evident to the commission that although prisoners who participate in research are informed and they do so freely, the conditions of social and economic deprivation in which they live compromise their freedom.[10]

This statement totally disregards the fact that almost all research that is done on humans is done under some form of constraint. The person dying of cancer or leukemia would not engage in activities "were they stronger or in better circumstances." What makes the prisoner under more constraint than the person dying of leukemia? Convicts are no more limited while prisoners of their own situation than the poor and the ill. The person dying of leukemia who is willing to undergo a dangerous and still unproven procedure in hopes of saving his or her own life is under much tighter constraints and under more severe duress.

There is no free choice in anything in life without some constraint, whether it be physical, psychological, or social. If a prisoner is competent and if the reason for incarceration is valid and not the result of a miscarriage of justice, then his informed consent within the constraints of his incarceration is as acceptable as is the informed consent of someone living within the constraints of their illness. This holds true unless we consider all prisoners as simply victims of society. Such thinking can lead to absurd conclusions. Free choice is always free choice within constraints.

Prisoners want to participate in experimentation for various reasons, but primarily for financial gain. This has been discussed by former prison inmate and research participant Frank Hatfield.[11] The income serves to provide items within the prison. Increased monies in prison also act as a cooling agent. There is less likely to be fighting over simple items when money is more freely available. Prison violence is diminished under these circumstances. Increased income also helps the prisoners maintain contact with the outside world, especially near Christmas time and the beginning of school vacations, when prisoners are eager to earn money to send home to their families. Some keep up their union dues so they have a better chance of getting a job when they get out. Money saved in prison may be of help in starting a new life when released. It is very rare that there are significant provisions for a prisoner at the time of his discharge. As a result and as expressed by John I. Arnold,

It is a fairly common consensus inside the prison that a return to crime, at least briefly, is the only way to manage during the early discharge period. This is often contrary to their real desires. To whatever degree money may diminish the pressures on a newly discharged inmate to commit a crime, the payment for participation in medical research should be considered as a possible help in crime prevention.[12]

Aside from the monetary gain there are also other factors such as a desire to do something for others, both on a purely altruistic basis and perhaps to satisfy some underlying sense of guilt. There may also be hope that doing good for someone else may be taken into consideration at parole hearings. In addition, participation in medication studies leads to extensive general physical examinations, which are much more thorough than the usual examinations a prisoner receives. Finally, participation in a human experimental program may give the prisoner a sense of purpose. Hatfield expresses this dynamic very well:

> Well-meaning people, who have never been in prison, seem to feel that they know what is best for convicts. I disagree. Men in prison have few material resources and are denied many aspects of human dignity. Those few opportunities they do have should not be taken away against their wishes unless society is prepared to offer a meaningful alternative.[13]

In regard to the rights of prisoners, society can, if it wishes, pass laws restricting any and all rights from someone who has committed a crime—even mandating capital punishment for shoplifting. But in spite of a common sense of vengefulness, reasonable people and reasonable societies tend to tailor the punishment to fit the crime with the prime thought being to deter others from committing the crime, to protect society, and to rehabilitate the criminal. In our approach to this problem we have removed certain rights, such as freedom, but those rights that have not been specifically removed remain intact within the established framework. Prisoners have the right to food, to read, to exercise, and to have limited contact with the outside world. Incarceration does not mean the abdication of all rights of the individual except the rights of his or her physical freedom and the right to disobey rules of imprisonment. Dr. Donald Seldin[14] stressed the right to participate in human experimentation programs within the general penumbra of human rights that remain inherent even for prisoners unless specifically denied by law. The principle of the Ninth Amendment is that any rights that are not specifically limited must be considered free. This concept should hold true inside as well as outside of prison.

The major flaw in the national commission's report was the result of the desire to reach a unanimous decision.[15] By doing so, a sharp separation between the purely ethical issues and the pragmatic problems of performing experiments upon prisoners became blurred. It would have been much wiser and more just had the commission made a clear-cut decision to validate a prisoner's right to participate in a properly formulated and executed research program, and then had demanded that every research program be more rigidly evaluated and controlled. There should have been a sharp separation between the pragmatic aspects of human experimentation and the ethical issues. Instead, as Branson suggests, "Their thinking seemed more influenced by . . . their assessment of the empirical condition of prisons."[16] It is possible that a more detached approach to the problem would have led to a demand for better management of experimentation rather than a ban on many types of experiments. The American Correctional Association made a similar error: "The authority which authorizes or permits prisoners to become subjects of human experimentation ignores his historic obligation as a custodian to protect and safely keep those for whom he assumes a legal responsibility."[17]

That legal responsibility is to see that the prisoner is not mistreated while in custody, which includes protecting him or her from *improper* experimentation, but that does not mean to mistreat the prisoner by removing the right to participate in *proper* experiments and to prevent gaining monetary strength so that life after prison may be less frightening. The American Correctional Association has thrown out the kettle with the soup.

The national commission's contention that research should not be conducted unless there are compelling reasons to involve prisoners[18] ignores the compelling nature of a prisoner's poverty, need for income, and the desire for a sense of self-respect. As a result of the arguments presented by those who oppose experimentation on prisoners, the national commission recommended that,

> Prisoners should not be subjects of research that is unrelated to their status as prisoners and is of no benefit to them (e.g., drug testing, research involving infectious diseases) unless there is an important social and scientific need and there are compelling reasons for involving prisoners in research. This recommendation was followed by the ruling that nontherapeutic research would not be permitted at all unless it involves no more than minimal risk and is designed to study the possible causes, effects and processes of incarceration, or the nature of prisons as institutional structures and of prisoners as incarcerated persons.[19]

What we are discussing are the ethical principles involved, the validity of performing proper experimentation on prisoners, not the inequities or inadequacies of a research program.

If experimentation in prisons cannot be done properly, it should not be performed, not because it is on a prisoner, but only because it cannot be done properly. To remove the opportunity to participate in human experimentation may be considered unwarranted restriction of activities. This restriction is not part of the punishment for which the person is in prison. It may be considered an additional and therefore illegal punishment. This would not only be unfair to the prisoner, but would be a loss to the common good of society.

FETAL EXPERIMENTATION

The problem of fetal experimentation is most difficult to discuss due to the question of consent. Throughout this work, I have attempted to remain consistent in regard to the consent of incompetent persons regardless of the reason for their incompetence, or the stage of life. To remain consistent, the reasonable substituted judgment standard, as discussed in chapter 4, must again apply.

In the following discussion the assumption is made that the proposed research program is valid scientifically and will be well performed, controlled, supervised, and evaluated by a research committee.

In regard to fetal experimentation, one faction believes that experiments on fetuses and children should only be considered if the results of the research may benefit the research subjects themselves. A second faction, exemplified by Richard McCormick,[20] suggests that even nontherapeutic experimentation is acceptable if it involves minimal or negligible risk on the basis that there is a moral obligation to do so under the rubric of the common good.

If the approach to nontherapeutic experiments on the young is looked at simply as a means to an end, then it becomes a dehumanizing act of misusing people, and a callous approach to personhood. On the other hand, if there is no risk or discomfort and reasonable grounds for assuming consent, then allowing participation in the experiment is to enable one to satisfy a moral obligation to do good.

First, it is apparent that people generally wish to feel they have contributed to society and that their obligations to do good have been fulfilled, that whatever moral debt they owe to society has been paid. This probably holds true for most competent people, and very reasonably may be assumed to be the desire or potential desire of an incompetent person regardless of age. Therefore, one may assume that an incompetent person would, if competent, not only wish to satisfy an obligation but would wish to do good even in the absence of an obligation.

The problem is, then, to establish parameters guiding such research programs. As described in chapter 1, one need not do good if the danger or distress of doing good is unacceptable. Under these circumstances, it is obvious that any experimentation that would not be of value to the subject and that may even remotely endanger the life or health of a normal intrauterine person or child would be unacceptable.

But what if the fetus is scheduled for abortion? Is experimentation permissible then and can reasonable substituted judgment be obtained to allow organs to be harvested for transplantation purposes? As expressed by pediatrician Eugene Diamond:

> One need not approve of abortion in order to allow the disposal of the tissues of the child who is dead as a result of the abortion. One need not approve of murder in order to allow the murder victim's body to be autopsied or his organs be donated.[21]

Is experimentation warranted if the decision to abort has already been made? It is mandatory in such a discussion that we keep separate the abortion issue from the use of fetal tissue. Regardless of how we may feel about abortion, at the time the abortion is decided upon, the ethical factors concerning use of fetal tissue come into play.

Many of us carry attached to our driver's licenses an

authorization for removal of kidneys or corneas if we are ever in a fatal accident. Many if not most people would allow organs to be removed at the time of death if we knew that such a donation may save another's life or help enhance another's health. On this same basis, reasonable substituted judgment suggests that an incompetent person, fetus or older, may also consent to organ procurement under such circumstances. To remain consistent, it appears that we must again ask the question: What would that patient wish to do if competent and aware of the circumstances?

It would be inconsistent to assume that I, as an adult who already has consigned my corneas and kidneys to others at the time of my death, would not be willing to do the same at any time of death. Would not the abortus, even though the abortion was not accidental, but deliberate, and not for the purpose of obtaining fetal tissue, through reasonable substituted judgment "think" in a similar fashion? Therein lies the probable validity of use of fetal tissue for transplantation purposes.

Let us discuss the ethical aspects in more detail. Fetal tissue has been used in experimental studies for many years. The potential value of these studies cannot be accurately measured, but it is enough to know that the knowledge gained would be good for society. That "good" obligates and grants society the right to ask to use fetal tissue, not necessarily the right to use it. The obligation of society to seek fetal tissue for transplantation and other studies reflects the factor of beneficence toward those who may benefit, and since there are potentially many who may benefit, the factor of common good also enters the scene. This must be balanced against autonomy in the form of consent for both mother and fetus. Nonmaleficence is not pertinent since abortion is already a given. Therefore, it is not a question of harm to the fetus. Nonmaleficence as well as beneficence toward the fetus would become pertinent if one encouraged conception for the purpose of obtaining fetal tissue that would harm the fetus. To do so would be to do harm. Henry Greely expresses it this way: "To use that tissue is to treat the fetus as nothing but a medical product and the uterus as a factory. It would demean the potential or actual humanity of the fetus."[22] This does not necessarily apply to the recent episode when a desperate family decided to have a baby in order to obtain blood marrow to save their older child. The donor infant was not harmed in the process.

Depending upon whether the abortus or soon-to-be abortus is considered a person or not would determine whether consideration is given primarily to fetal autonomy or to the woman's autonomy. Under the principle of autonomy, at minimum there would have to be proper consent from the mother and proper respect in the handling of fetal tissue, at maximum, consent from both (using reasonable substituted judgment for the fetus) would be necessary. But since abortion is a given, fetal consent may be assumed to be granted.

Both the ethical and the complex political issues concerning fetal tissue transplantation were discussed by Annas and Elias[23] and the ethical aspects were reviewed by the Stanford University Medical Center Committee on Ethics, chaired by Dr. Henry Greely.[24] The following guidelines have been proposed by the Stanford University committee:

> Human fetal tissue should generally be treated with the respect given cadavers, and its use should be governed by the same legal rules.
>
> Women who undergo induced abortions should not be allowed to benefit directly from the subsequent medical use of the fetal tissue, through payment for it, through the reimbursement of expenses connected with the abortion, or in any other manner. The National Organ Transplantation Act should be amended to cover human fetal tissue—whether used for transplantation or any other medical purpose—and to exclude abortion-related expenses from its definition of permissible reimbursement.

Because of the possibility that a conflict of interest might affect their advice to patients about abortion, medical personnel who perform induced abortions should not be allowed any direct benefit from the subsequent use of the fetal tissue.

The proper medical use of fetal tissue from spontaneous abortions and from abortions induced because of risk to the mother's life is ethically unobjectionable.

The use of tissue from fetuses aborted for the specific purpose of donating that tissue seems ethically impermissible. . . .

Subject to these conditions, human fetal tissue can be used ethically for medical research and treatment.[25]

Continuous research on humans is mandatory if we are to improve mental and physical health and prolong life. Our problem is to do it as safely as possible, without coercion, and with honest informed consent. Aside from the above, problems include the compulsive drive to receive grants, to fund research programs, and the immense pressure placed upon academic scientists to obtain grants not only to help their research but to supply the academic institution with additional resources, since a large portion of each grant is appropriated by the institution. This academic pressure to publish or perish occasionally results in premature or inaccurate scientific conclusions.

NOTES

1. Hans Jonas, in *Experimentation with Human Beings,* Jay Katz, ed. (New York: Russell Sage Foundation, 1972), p. 148.

2. Jay Katz, ed., *Experimentation with Human Beings* (New York: Russell Sage Foundation, 1972), p. 121.

3. Ibid., p. 48.

4. Ibid., p. 49.

5. Ibid.

6. Ibid., p. 51.

7. National Commission for the Protection of Human Subjects of Biomedical and Behavioral Research, DHEW Publication no. [OS] 76-131, 1976.

8. Ibid., p. 7.

9. Edmond Cahn, in Katz, *Experimentation with Human Beings,* p. 1041.

10. National Commission, p. 6.

11. Frank Hatfield, "Prison Research: The View from Inside," *Hastings Center Report* 7, no. 1 (Feruary 1977): 11–12.

12. Katz, *Experimentation with Human Beings,* p. 1023.

13. Hatfield, "Prison Research: The View from Inside," p. 12.

14. Roy Branson, "Prison Research," *Hastings Center Report* 7, no. 1 (February 1977): 15–21, p. 17.

15. Ibid., p. 19.

16. Ibid., p. 19.

17. Ibid. Position statement of American Correctional Association, p. 16.

18. Ibid., p. 18.

19. National Commission Summary of Activities, Reading no. 1612, Institute of Society, Ethics and the Life Sciences, Hastings-On-Hudson, New York (May 17, 1978).

20. Richard A. McCormick, "Proxy Consent in the Experimental Situation," *Perspectives in Biology and Medicine* 18 (1974): 14.

21. Eugene F. Diamond, "Redefining the Issues in Fetal Experimentation," *Journal American Medical Association* 236, no. 3 (July 16, 1976): 281–83, p. 281.

22. H. T. Greely et al., "The Ethical Use of Human Fetal Tissue in Medicine," *The New England Journal of Medicine* 320, no. 16 (April 20, 1989): 1093–96.

23. G. J. Annas and S. Elias, "The Politics of Transplantation of Human Fetal Tissue," *The New England Journal of Medicine* 320, no. 16 (April 20, 1989): 1079–82.

24. Greely, "The Ethical Use of Human Fetal Tissue in Medicine."

25. Ibid.

10

The Ethics of Medical Triage

Allocation and Rationing of Health Care

This chapter will not deal with the details of triage but with the ethical problems related to it. The countless ramifications of triage are well summarized by Roger W. Evans.[1]

Triage is a French word for sorting, picking out, or sifting. It is a system designed to produce the greatest benefit from limited resources. The term became prominent during World War I, when ambulance drivers devised a system of priorities as to which wounded soldiers would receive treatment first. The crux of the issue was determining who could be sent back to battle most easily. This meant that those who were seriously injured and unable to fight were left to the end and sometimes left to die. There were simply not enough physicians, nurses, hospital personnel or facilities to treat all patients simultaneously. Some had to wait. Under the doctrine of fairness, people should have been treated according to the principle of first-come-first-served, or on the basis of treating those who would die if not treated. However, the doctrine of common good gave society's war effort first priority, so treatment of those who would not be able to return to battle was delayed.

With full appreciation that of all areas of human condition health is usually held most precious, especially during times of illness, our society has attempted to bring adequate health care to all. This has been done with such vigor that some now consider health care a fundamental right. It is not. But that does not mean that society is not obligated to treat the ill.

The concept that no one who needs treatment should go untreated is admirable and certainly every effort should be made to accomplish that end, but to assume that people have a right to health care must be challenged. The individual has only the *right to seek health care* and society has *the moral obligation to try to provide health care*. This obligation goes beyond the mere force of popular vote or desire. The beneficence principal mandates that all citizens have access to adequate health care.

If we appreciate the immensity of potential medical costs, we must realize that it is physically and economically impossible to satisfy all medical demands utilizing all contemporary knowledge and technology for the aged, chronically ill, disabled, mentally ill, mentally handicapped, as well as acute illnesses, even if we were to ignore preventive medicine and care of the malnourished.

Psychological and psychiatric aid alone for all those who could benefit from it would demand a massive increase in the number of mental health professionals and the expense would be overwhelming.

Associated with the issue of equal access to health care is that of access to equal quality of health care. The human condition is one of differences in abilities, positions, functions, living locations, opportunities, and accessibilities to each and every aspect of opportunity. To ignore this fact is to ignore reality. As it is impossible for each person to live in the most beautiful home overlooking the sea, so it is impossible for each person to have access to the finest of medical care. There is a limited number of talented and accomplished physicians. As there are inequalities in artistic capabilities so are there inequalities in medical and surgical capabilities. The brilliant and talented are not commonplace in any field. Economics aside, the mere fact that only a small percentage of physicians are highly accomplished automatically condemns the public to unequal medical care whether they like to think of it in those terms or not. The wealthy can seek out the best, the poor can hope for the best. Equal access to the *best* of health care is a destructive misconception. Equality of health care is neither possible nor necessary. What is necessary is access to good quality of care. Equality of health care does not exist in any nation of the world regardless of resources or standard of living. Robert Hudson states it well:

> The pursuit of equal-health-for-all will be a disservice to all, because equal health is no more attainable than equal justice. . . . Neither ideal is ultimately realizable in view of our system of personal and economic freedom, to say nothing of the harsh reality of unequal genetic endowment.[2]

The maximum that we can hope and work for is to improve the pattern of each person's life, to provide good care, to strive that each may have the finest in life and to know that the goal is beyond reach.

The President's Commission stated that,

> Patients, health care professionals, and institutions, and society at large must . . . choose the uses to which . . . resources will be put. The choices require comparing health care expenditures with other areas of public and private spending as well as choices within the health care budget— between treatment and research; between restorative steps for those already ill and preventive steps for those who may be at risk; among different age groups, diseases, treatment settings and so forth.[3]

The commission was unable to establish a clear-cut path. It did not find clear principles upon which to manage triage except to consider the principle of equity, which is in itself difficult to delineate:

> The principles of equity do not create a "right" to health care equal to all the care that some people may obtain for themselves. . . . Rather, equity requires that people have access to adequate levels of care and that cost of care be fairly distributed.[4]

When we apply the concept of triage to health care we must appreciate its two major components, allocation and rationing. Allocation refers to how much money society wishes to budget for health care. Rationing refers to the selection of which patients are to have access to limited medical facilities.

ALLOCATION

The more we allocate funds for health the less the need for rationing. Since the need to ration health services should be reduced as much as possible, society must make hard choices and decide how much to allocate for health care and still take care of the other aspects of social living, e.g., education, social welfare, and defense. The degree of support each segment of society can expect is obviously a subject for debate. We must therefore reexamine our values and set our priorities in light of limited resources.

How do we weigh relative needs and harms during the allocation process? How do we decide which patient group should be more or less favored? Where would greater harm be produced by the limitation of funds? Should we limit funds necessary to care for victims of Alzheimer's disease, restrict funds necessary to provide dental care for all children, or reduce the funds necessary to supply the blind with seeing-eye dogs? This ethical dilemma, which demands that we balance harms, becomes even more complex when we have to balance health needs with the need to control acid rain and water pollution, let alone improve housing for the poor and homeless and supply food for the hungry.

Great Britain, in its attempt to control costs, prevented the proliferation of expensive computerized tomography (CT) and magnetic resonance imaging (MRI) equipment, and has deliberately limited the formation of dialysis units in hospitals.

There are approximately ten thousand people each year who are in a persistent vegetative state at a minimum annual cost of over $100,000. That accounts for $1 billion for care of patients who, the vast majority through reasonable substituted judgment, would not want to exist in that hopeless state. Aside from the continuing anguish in the hearts of family, is that economic burden on the family and state warranted? Any decision to cease active treatment of these patients is loaded with anguish.

The cardiac bypass procedure now so commonly performed in the United States is rapidly expanding throughout the world. The cost of each operation is approximately $75,000. Not all who would benefit from this surgery can receive it. What will happen when a practical mechanical heart and lung are designed? The economic burden of such technology, if made available to all who need and desire it, would be immense.

We may have to reevaluate other specific issues. For example, should problems of infertility be subsidized? Is this financial effort beyond society's obligation? In Massachusetts alone cost estimates of this problem are $5.5 million to $100 million. Does the degree of beneficence warrant this degree of expense?

The problem of allocating funds for research must also be faced. How prudent is our use of these funds? Ethical considerations demand a careful evaluation of what is best for the common good. The federal government has already spent over $160 million of limited research funds in the attempt to develop a totally implantable heart. Policy decisions regarding the use of these funds must more seriously consider endeavors that may have greater significance than the development of artificial hearts. Should such funds be directed toward the development of efficient contraceptive techniques to help control the massive influx of unwanted children in our poverty areas? Is the need to develop an artificial heart in order to prolong life anywhere nearly as urgent as the need to control population, to feed the hungry, and to treat the diseased who are already here? Research for contraception and programs to upgrade the standard of living are certainly not as dramatic as research on the creation of an artificial heart. But where is the greater good? Are we being influenced by the romance of fancy technology? It may be time for our scientific review boards to reestablish priorities. This may be an important effort not only for the common good of our nation but for all nations.

This brings up the important but unpleasant realization that patients with different diseases could reasonably perceive each other as rivals for care or research efforts.

Only the public, by open discussion of allocations, can make these value judgments and broad decisions. Attempts to give preferential funding to one type of patient at the expense of other patients is apt to provoke public uproar. But that uproar may have to be confronted unless society is willing to accept the financial burden to care for all health problems. In the decision-making process for the allocation of funds the most pertinent ethical factors are the common good and nonmaleficence. During this process society must decide how to produce the least harm, or the direction in which lies the greatest common good. The factors of autonomy and beneficence assume relatively unimportant positions in allocation decisions, although beneficence may be used as the positive variation of nonmaleficence.

RATIONING

Rationing is and has always been a fact of life. Not all people have or ever had equal opportunity to obtain the finest of health care. The question is not whether rationing exists, but how we can make it less distasteful.

In every hospital emergency room as well as at the scene of accidents where several people have been hurt, patients are triaged. Time and service are rationed. Those patients who are at risk of dying are given first priority.

It is routine practice in the management of hospital intensive care units (ICUs), where the number of beds are limited, to evaluate patients as to who may be removed from the intensive care unit when a new patient arrives in critical condition. How do I tell the patient, who just two hours previously was told that she will have to remain in the ICU to be certain that complications do not occur, that she will now have to be moved because a more seriously ill patient needs that space? The inevitable response is, "Why me?" A decision is made independent of the patient's wishes and sometimes contrary to the wishes of the attending physician, who is primarily concerned with his or her own patient, not someone else's. How do we balance the harms that ensue when one person in need is given preference over another person? When facilities are limited, on what basis do we determine which person should be given access to them? These questions are frequently resolved by the director of the ICU, who has no conflict of interest. The patient in less need would be sent to the regular nursing area with the full realization that by doing so the risk of catastrophe is now higher for that patient, but still not as high as the risk of catastrophe for the newly arrived patient if placed in the regular nursing area. This is triage. The potential harm to each patient has to be balanced. This is purely a medical judgment.

Rationing and containment of costs are interwoven. Unless the public increases the amount of money dedicated to health care, physicians, families, and patients will have to make unpleasant and sometimes heartbreaking decisions. Triage through cost containment will eventually become much more obvious than it is at the present time. By the year 2000 it is anticipated that there will be nearly 32 million people over the age of sixty-five, which is more than 12 percent of the total population. This age group will demand a great deal of medical care. The burden of supplying that medical care will fall upon the resources of the younger generation. Harsh decisions will have to be made. Many will be hurt, but the federal government or third-party insurers must face this dilemma regardless of how onerous the choices may be. Nicholas Rescher suggests that if we refuse to accept this responsibility, finding it arrogant or odious, future patient selection will either be random or will favor the rich and the well-connected over the poor and powerless.[5]

There are four factors that compound the problem. They include population growth, population aging, the increasing prevalence of chronic diseases, disabilities as a result of better medical care, and the continuing development of new technology such as new imaging devices and the ability to replace arthritic joints.

There are several approaches to this problem. First, designate medical parameters, such as age, that would automatically limit, at least for the elderly, the extent to which illnesses will be treated. Great Britain utilized age alone when it decided that payments would not be made for renal dialysis therapy given to patients over sixty years of age. The federal government spends about $2 billion per year for the renal dialysis program. Approximately 15 to 20 percent of renal dialysis patients are unable to lead useful or functioning lives. A valid and pointed question is presented by Dr. Arnold S. Relman, who asks whether money spent on an eighty-year-old patient who is barely surviving would not be better spent in other areas of medical research.[6]

Stanford University utilized a similar approach when it applied the age bracket criteria to triage cardiac patients. Physicians decided that heart transplants would be limited to those below the age of fifty. The pros and cons of using age as a determining factor in cost containment are discussed at length by John Kilner,[7] of the Asbury Theological Seminary. Daniel Callahan suggests that, "After a person has lived out a natural life span, medical care should no longer be oriented to resisting death . . . it would normally be expected by late seventies or early eighties."[8]

A second approach, one that most physicians would prefer, is to consider the patient's physiological age as a much better parameter regarding treatment than chronological age. The eighty-five-year-old "young" vital person with temporary renal disease would certainly be considered a candidate for dialysis and be treated more aggressively than the fifty-year-old frail patient who is already senile. Chronological age per se should not be a factor in the discussion of cost containment. Parameters such as life expectancy, general status of health, and the logistics of health-care delivery are pertinent factors within this approach to triage.

A third approach would combine medical parameters with social criteria, such as family role and one's value to society. According to Nicholas Rescher:

> All things being equal, the mother of four must take priority over a middle-aged bachelor. An egalitarian society may be reluctant to decide between a brilliant surgeon and a skillful laborer. But could not a case be made for society choosing a surgeon who in turn would be able to save many other lives?[9]

I can easily accept Rescher's first value judgment, but I cannot accept the concept of relative value to society. To place relative values on people because of their social position would be dehumanizing and humiliating. It would officially stratify society, which is contrary to everything we hold true regarding each person's sense of worth. But I must admit that if only one kidney were available for transplantation, as a physician, I doubt that I would approve granting that kidney to a child molester in prison as opposed to a school teacher. I do not doubt that regardless of what laws may be passed, at the microrationing level, although it may be distasteful, the decision-making process will include three factors: first-come-first-served, the potential quality of life, and, to a much lesser degree, the social value to society. All three will at times play a role in the decision as to who will (or will not) receive a needed organ. In a survey of renal dialysis units, Kilner exposed the fact that medical and social factors were significant in rationing renal dialysis when the demand was greater than the physical resources necessary to treat.[10] This decision-making process is not without an emotional burden that the medical team must live with.

Another avenue would be for insurers to ration/allocate resources by managing payments. This can be accomplished by specifying which hospitals, which procedures, and even which physicians and surgeons will be compensated for health care. The potential success of heart transplant programs and other highly team-oriented and expensive procedures warrants such a consideration for two reasons. One is simple fiscal responsibility, and the other would be to help concentrate highly specialized and expensive activities in major centers where the volume of cases would enhance greater expertise. But although financial control of resources may act as a rationing force, it will not speak to the question as to who is to receive the needed care. From a practical point of view, the wealthy and powerful will probably be more able to obtain the care they need, so that medical triage is primarily aimed at those less fortunate economically. We cannot restrict the right of someone to seek medical care, nor can we restrict the right of those practitioners who wish to practice outside of a controlled, tax-supported facility. But within such a facility, rules may be set that could restrict the use of limited resources according to preset medical parameters.

There are some cost-containment measures that have strong ethical implications independent of the economic aspect, since the present system may produce harm to patients. These measures may be for the good of all patients and therefore for the common good.

A significant number of surgeries are performed by doctors who have not had thorough surgical training. Insurance companies and governmental funding agencies should consider paying the costs of surgery only when performed by qualified surgeons* (unless there are extenuating medical circumstances and except for minor office procedures). This would lead patients to more expert medical care, reduce the number of unnecessary and ineptly performed surgeries and the complications arising from inept surgeries. It would lead to better utilization of more qualified surgeons, who would subsequently develop a better body of experience to the benefit of patients. This does not imply that all nonqualified surgeons are inept, nor that qualified surgeons do not do inept or unnecessary surgery, but as a general rule it appears wiser to have surgery performed by those who have at least completed the prescribed amount and type of training necessary.

Patients would still have the right to have surgery performed by any nonqualified surgeon who may legally do any type of surgery that he or she feels capable of performing. But, under the circumstances, the patient would be completely responsible for any surgical or hospital expenses.

Such a program would pragmatically improve medical care while decreasing medical expenses. At the same time, qualified surgeons who also do family practice to augment their income would be more likely to transfer such patients to where they more properly belong—the family physicians.

---

*A member of the American College of Surgeons or its equivalent, or a physician with at least ten years experience as a surgeon.

It would benefit patients both medically and financially if the number of procedures they are exposed to could be reduced. This may be accomplished by eliminating physicians' potential financial conflicts of interest. When physicians own part of hospitals, extended care facilities, pharmacies, laboratories, and especially imaging equipment, there is an inclination to overuse these facilities. This is not only immoral but extremely costly to society. Except for certain specialties and unusual circumstances these investments should be considered unacceptable to funding agencies. This may best be controlled if the funding agencies, as prudent trustees of public funds, demand that all such facilities reveal their ownership prior to any payment of funds.

Professor of Surgery George Dunlop[11] suggests that the number of blood tests as well as other procedures would probably be reduced if the cost of each test was printed on the test requisition form and on the reporting forms so that interns, residents, and attending physicians become more aware of the expense factor when ordering these tests. This is independent of the need to reduce the number of tests and procedures done in anticipation of a possible malpractice suit.

An unpleasant area involving the ethics of cost containment and rationing involves the unceasing traffic, between nursing homes and acute hospitals, of senile, terminal, or near-terminal patients. One physician specializing in the care of patients in convalescent homes put it this way:

> For these patients, even the best result would only let them return to the extended care facility they came from. There, some of these patients become agitated and physically combative, sometimes injuring themselves or other patients or their caretakers. They will have to be physically or chemically restrained; . . . others will nod away with complete withdrawal from everything around them, either confined to bed or strapped in wheelchairs. Many will need NG (nasogastric) tube feedings. Many will soil themselves

and their bedclothes night and day. The status of many will inevitably worsen. Then they will go back to an acute hospital for treatment of recurring fecal impactions, hip fractures, sepsis, sudden falls in hemoglobin, pneumonia, congestive failure, strokes, TIAs* and other conditions.[12]

This pattern of care involving very elderly, incapacitated and often severely senile patients in extended care facilities, flouts their often-stated desire not to prolong life. These actions can be measured in billions of dollars aside from the prolongation of the patient's anguish and the family's distress.

To alter the situation, patients in extended care facilities who fall into this category should be identified. Discussions should be held with the medical director of the facility, the director of nursing, the family, and, if possible, the patient. A decision should be reached after open discussion and a program outlined regarding the question of whether transfer to an acute hospital for the prolongation of life is to be considered if medical problems arise, or whether comfort should be the only goal. Such information, necessary to help stop administering unwanted medical care and at the same time conserve billions of dollars, is now mandated by law. "Directives to the Physician" and to the facility are required to be available to all patients and their families as of December 1, 1991, in all hospitals and extended care facilities. Wanzer believes it is

especially important that nursing homes require a regular review of patient preferences, with each patient's physician taking responsibility for ensuring that such information is obtained and documented. In the case of patients who lack decision-making capacity, surrogate decision makers should be identified and consulted appropriately.[13]

---

*Transient ischemic attacks.

Is it ever warranted to force-feed a permanently senile patient by the insertion of a nasogastric tube, a procedure not uncommon in nursing homes? Should those who do not wish to live longer and those who are so incompetent that life has no significant meaning, be treated to prolong life? Therapy to relieve discomfort must never be withheld, but to institute therapy to prolong unwanted life is certainly questionable. Reasonable substituted judgment, respect for autonomy, and the requirements of nonmaleficence would deem otherwise.

NOTES

1. Roger W. Evans, "Health Care Technology and the Inevitability of Resource Allocation and Rationing Decisions, Part 1," *JAMA: Journal American Medical Association* 249, no. 15 (April 15, 1983): 2047-52; " Part 2," *JAMA* 249, no. 16 (April 22, 1983): 2208-19.

2. Robert P. Hudson, "How Real Is Our Reverence for Life," *Prism* (June 1975): 19-20.

3. The President's Commission for the Study of Ethical Problems in Medicine and Biomedical and Behavioral Research, "Summing Up" (March 1983), p. 72.

4. Ibid., p. 74.

5. Nicholas Rescher, "Whose Life Should We Save When the Technology Is Scarce?" *Los Angeles Times* (March 10, 1986).

6. Arnold Relman, *Newsweek* (August 31, 1981): p. 54.

7. John F. Kilner, "Age as a Basis for Allocating Life Saving Medical Resources: An Ethical Analysis," *Journal of Health, Politics, Policy, and Law* 13, no. 3 (Fall 1988): 405-40.

8. Daniel Callahan, "Terminating Treatment: Age as a Standard," *Hastings Center Report* 17, no. 5 (October-November 1987): 25.

9. Rescher, "Whose Life Should We Save. . . ."

10. John F. Kilner, "Selecting Patients When Resources are Limited," *American Journal of Public Health* 78, no. 2 (February 1988): 144-47.

11. George Dunlop, M.D., personal communication, 1990.

12. Howard Caplan, "We Cannot Afford to Prolong So Many Hopeless Lives," *Medical Economics for Surgeons* (February 1983): 30–32.

13. Sidney Wanzer et al., "The Physician's Responsibility toward Hopelessly Ill Patients," *New England Journal of Medicine* (March 30, 1989): 845.

Summary

The foundation of this book lies within its first chapter, "A Concept of Ethics." There has been so much written about medical ethics, and from so many different points of view, that the ethical waters have been muddied. The persistent attempt to invoke religious concepts in the ethical dilemmas of our secular society, right as they may well be within their own framework, has added to the confusion. The rigidity within fervent religiosity does not readily permit nor accept contrary views of ethics. I have made a specific attempt to set forth what I believe to be a reasonable approach to ethics devoid of religious bias. As a result, four factors are identified that must be considered in the evaluation of every ethical situation: nonmaleficence, freedom, the common good, and beneficence.

I hope that I have avoided falling into a specific category or school of ethics. All too often labels such as "utilitarianism" are confining, inadequate, and incorrect.

The subsequent chapters are primarily constructed to portray the applicability of the four moral factors and the importance of the hierarchy developed at the outset. These moral factors are equally applicable to all other ethical problems in medicine, including genetic engineering, psychosurgery, and the management of the AIDS patient.

The chapters that discuss the doctor-patient relationship, the right of self-determination, and suicide primarily stress the right of people to decide what is best for themselves, the right of competent patients to control their own destiny, and the need to understand that the physician is the agent of the patient. The chapters on abortion, the tragic newborn, euthanasia, human experimentation, and triage emphasize the importance of balancing the four moral factors in situations where individual rights may more obviously conflict with societal rights and obligations.

In the discussions there may appear to be a sense of detachment, a feeling that decisions are made in an emotional vacuum on purely philosophical or legal grounds. This would be an unfortunate impression. Emotional turmoil is always present within the doctor-patient-family relationship when in intimate contact with illness and especially impending death. This emotional struggle cannot be ignored. It is important to realize that decisions regarding life and death may be made on a purely emotional basis or within a more disciplined format. It is not always a question of which approach is right or wrong; it may be a question of what the parties involved can live with in later years. Although we should think dispassionately, we cannot divorce ourselves from the emotional aspects of these decisions. Remorse, whether rational or not, can be devastating, but its impact is usually exaggerated. Life almost always resumes its "normal" course if the decision is based upon cautious and disciplined reasoning.

A final word. Much of the debate surrounding the issues of abortion, suicide, and euthanasia have nothing to do with ethics, but flourish and flounder in the political sea.

Appendix A

Discussion of Mastery*

Mastery speaks of the ability to reach a specific goal—to have control—to win. The biological advantage of achieving mastery is an integral part of the survival and procreation of the most adaptive or stronger organism.

Mastery involves stressful behavior patterns. Phylogenetically it is related to self-preservation as seen when the more dominant animal takes first opportunity to satisfy hunger, as well as to species preservation as part of the pattern of sexual forwardness against competitors for the mate and hesitance of the sexual partner. Within this forwardness is doubt of success, which mingles with the sexual hunger. This doubt produces tension and anxiety which subsequently become intimately enmeshed with sensuousness. Mastery, like curiosity, serves both the self and species preservation.

It is reasonable to assume that in the drive toward mastery, in the competition for food and for mating, that, as with the phenomenon of curiosity, a feeling of pleasure slowly evolved to join whatever behavior would lead to the achievement of mastery. This pleasure would in turn encourage the formation of behavior to be masterful.

---

*See chapter 1, p. 29.

This close tie between tension and sensuality becomes, with learning, even more enmeshed and expanded. It may become so strongly allied that some seek most of their sexual satisfaction through stress and conflict.

Examples of mastery in the more primitive animal include the pecking order of chickens and the penile display action of the squirrel monkey. It is part of a behavior pattern that enhances survival of the stronger of the species and underscores the creation of an organism more apt to survive through the process of natural selection.

The phenomenon of mastery and the pleasure associated with it accounts, to some extent, for the pleasure obtained from the control of fear, the negation of insecurity, the establishment of order out of disorder, the recognition of that which was difficult to recognize, the sudden insight to the core of a dilemma, the solving of a complex problem, the concept of victory, climbing mountains, the achievement of power, the accumulation of wealth or material things, the control over personal inadequacies, the experience of the child who has successfully tied his shoes for the first time, and, as our behavior patterns become complex, even altruism and philanthropy with their unconscious feeling of mastery over people and events.[1]

The stance of human pride, as a reflection of mastery, is in many ways related to the strut and body tightness of the stud who wins his territory and his mare.

Mastery as a mechanism becomes a significant element in enhancing other mechanisms leaning toward pleasure. As we continue the process of gaining pleasure, regardless of what basic modality is brought into play, we not only gain what is expected but also gain an added dimension of pleasure through the mastery of achieving it. This is especially true whenever the thrust is *consciously* directed toward satisfying our desires.

There is therefore at least a two-fold basis for the development of pleasure under most circumstances: the primary source and the pleasure through mastery of gaining it.

It is reasonable to assume that through the process of learning and conditioning, the sense—the feeling—of mastery in itself subsequently becomes pleasurable through recall, without any further incident of mastery. The mere recall of mastery may become exciting. The strong ego is pleasurable.

However we modify or control the primitive brain with our massive cortex, the emotional substance of humankind remains a reflection of the primitive emotive stance. Hidden in the unconscious, the primitive emotional patterns underlie, to some extent, all human emotions. The development of more complex variations of emotional overtones, whether it be the taste of fine wine, the pleasure of music, the boxer smashing the face of his opponent, or watching the sun filter through deep woodlands, does not imply totally different mechanisms, but only derivatives of the basic pleasures associated with sensuousness, curiosity, and mastery.

NOTE

1. John Bowlby, *Attachment and Loss. Vol. I, Attachment* (New York: Basic Books, Inc., 1969), pp. 131–32.

Appendix B

Discussion of Privacy*

The word "privacy" is derived from the Latin *privatus,* meaning "not belonging to the state," or "not in public life." The historical impetus in the United States underlying the protection of privacy was to prevent undue police intrusions and to limit arbitrary government actions.

Privacy is derived from both the basic premise of autonomy and the factor of harm. The essence of autonomy lies in the ability to make a choice. To prevent free choice is to inflict harm. Privacy results from the choice to be left alone. It includes the right to choose to keep to oneself any and all information regarding his or her own person, actions, and thoughts; to prevent intrusion into one's physical being and property; and to choose to be left alone, isolated, untouched, and unknown (not to have one's affairs publicized).

The right to privacy, like all human rights, may be qualified. The problem of how and when to qualify this right again reflects the conflict between the right of an individual and the desire of "society" or of other individuals who may wish to intrude upon privacy. The demand for due process is the greatest protector of privacy.

---

*See chapter 4, p. 71.

Although the word "privacy" is not specifically mentioned in our Constitution, its presence, as an inherent part of freedom, is evident in both the Declaration of Independence and the Bill of Rights. The Declaration of Independence speaks of the "pursuit of happiness," which implies doing or not doing what we wish. This may well include the desire for privacy if we wish it. In the Constitution privacy is reflected to some degree in the First Amendment, which allows "the right of the people to peaceably assemble" in private if they so desire, as long as it is peaceful. The Third Amendment maintains the privacy of the home by prohibiting its use by the military without consent of the owners in time of peace, and only through due process in time of war. The Fourth Amendment again protects privacy by providing that, "The right of the people to be secure in their persons, houses, papers, and effects against unreasonable searches and seizures, shall not be violated, and no warrants shall issue, but upon probable cause, supported by oath or affirmation, and particularly describing the place to be searched and the persons or things to be seized." This amendment outlawed the concept of a general warrant that could so easily be abused at the expense of privacy.

The Fifth Amendment created a zone of privacy around the individual by declaring that no one "shall be compelled in any criminal case to be a witness against himself, nor be deprived of life, liberty, or property, without due process of law." The due process aspect solidified this privacy. The Fourteenth Amendment reaffirmed the due process clause by the statement that, "No State shall make or enforce any law which shall abridge the privileges or immunities of citizens of the United States; nor shall any State deprive any person of life, *liberty* or property, without due process of law" (emphasis added).

Privacy is also inherent within the intent of the Ninth Amendment, which states that, "The enumeration in the

Constitution of certain rights, shall not be construed to deny or disparage others retained by the people." This certainly can be applied to privacy, as a right reserved to the people.

The importance of privacy has been repeatedly emphasized by the United States Supreme Court. In 1891, the Court stressed that the right to privacy not only pertained to invasion of private surroundings, but also included the right to be left alone physically: "No right is held more sacred, or is more carefully guarded, by the common law, than the right of every individual to the possession and control of his own person, free from all restraint or interference by others, unless by clear and unquestionable authority of law."[1]

The matter of privacy against invasion of one's own physical being was again the issue when Judge Benjamin Cardozo stated that, "Every human being of adult years and sound mind has a right to determine what shall be done with his own body."[2] This statement speaks to the medical issues of abortion, surgery without consent, and suicide. It was reiterated in the *Natanson* v. *Kline* case: "Each man is considered to be master of his own body, and he may, if he be of sound mind, expressly prohibit the performance of life saving surgery, or other medical treatment."[3] And finally, in 1973, in the *Roe* v. *Wade* decision pertaining to abortion, the issue of physical privacy was again upheld. Privacy and personal freedom is expressed by the statement that, "The right of privacy . . . is broad enough to encompass a woman's decision whether or not to terminate her pregnancy."[4] But this was not an unqualified right, since specific requirements were outlined regulating how to perform an abortion during the third trimester.

Privacy in respect to one's surroundings, independent of one's own body, was emphasized in a case concerning wiretapping. In this situation, Justice Louis Brandeis in 1928 stated that the authors of the Constitution "knew that only a part of the pain, pleasure and satisfactions of life are to be found in material things. They sought to protect Americans in their beliefs, their thoughts, their emotions and their sensations." (They) "conferred, as against the government, the right to be let alone—the most comprehensive of rights and the right most valued by civilized men."[5]

This concept of Brandeis's was reemphasized by the Supreme Court and became legal precedent in 1967 in the *Katz* decision,[6] when the use of electronic listening devices outside the physical surroundings of the individual were considered a violation of privacy and unlawful under the Fourth Amendment.

Privacy was again stressed and broadened in 1965 when the Supreme Court prevented the government from interfering with the right of adults to procure and use contraceptive devices.[7] In this situation the question of invasion of person or property, self-incrimination, or unwanted publicity was not an issue.

When we ask under what circumstances society can invade an individual's privacy, we are implying that the factor of harm, benevolence, or the common good are pertinent factors, for only in the presence of one or all of these factors can the question even be posed.

What should our attitude be in regard to qualifying or invading privacy? We must establish which factors are pertinent and then weigh their importance against the abridgement of freedom. Our attitude should be that to infringe upon any element of freedom is undesirable and to be done only with the greatest trepidation.

As a result of our expanding population, our general sense of detachment from control, and our subsequent sense of dehumanization, our privacy has been slowly eroded. We must resist this trend and attempt to reestablish privacy's eminence. We erode our liberty through the outpouring of laws, executive orders, administrative regulations, and bureaucratic guidelines. Any rule or regulation that restricts liberty in any form must have strong justification, and must always be viewed as suspect.

The problem of control of the government and self-restraint by the government is difficult. Who or what institution of society must make that judgment? If society makes it, then who is to judge the judgment of society? One major problem is expressed by Professor Philip Kurland. He states that,

> The greatest, but not the exclusive problem of privacy is to question how to contain the government which is its own regulator. Here, as elsewhere we have turned to the courts.[8]

NOTES

1. *Union Pacific Railroad* v. *Botsford,* 141 U.S. 240 251 (1891).

2. *Schloendorff* v. *Society of New York Hospital,* 211 N.Y. 125 129–30,105 N.B. 92 93 (1914).

3. *Natanson* v. *Kline,* 186 Kan 393 406–7, 350 P2d 1093, 1104 (1960).

4. *Roe* v. *Wade,* 410 U.S. 116 (1973).

5. *Olmstead* v. *United States,* 277 U.S. 438, 378 (1928).

6. *Katz* v. *United States,* 389, U.S. 347, 350 (1967).

7. *Griswold* v. *Connecticut,* 381 U.S. 479 (1965).

8. Philip Kurland, "The Private I, Some Reflections on Privacy and the Constitution," *The University of Chicago Magazine* (Autumn 1976).

Appendix C

Example of Durable Power of Attorney

I, ___(name)___, do hereby designate and appoint: Name: _____ Address: _____ Telephone Number: _____ as my attorney-in-fact (agent) to make health-care decisions for me as authorized in this document.

GENERAL STATEMENT OF AUTHORITY GRANTED

If I become incapable of giving informed consent for health care decisions, I hereby grant to my agent full power and authority to make health care decisions for me, including the right to consent, refuse consent, or withdraw consent for any care, treatment service, or procedure to maintain, diagnose, or treat a physical or mental condition, and to receive and to consent for the release of medical information. I acknowledge that my attorney-in-fact fully understands my desire regarding my potential mental or physical health or death.

_____   _____
Witness   Signature

_____   _____
Date   Date

Appendix D

Recommendations Regarding Fetal Research

1. *Therapeutic research directed toward the fetus* may be conducted or supported, and should be encouraged, by the Secretary, DHEW,* provided such research (a) conforms to appropriate medical standards, (b) has received the informed consent of the mother, the father not dissenting, and (c) has been approved by existing review procedures with adequate provision for the monitoring of the consent process. (Adopted unanimously.)

2. *Therapeutic research directed toward the pregnant woman* may be conducted or supported, and should be encouraged, by the Secretary, DHEW, provided such research (a) has been evaluated for possible impact on the fetus, (b) will place the fetus at risk to the minimum extent consistent with meeting the health needs of the pregnant woman, (c) has been approved by existing review procedures with ade-

From *Research on the Fetus*, DHEW Publication No. (OS) 76-127 (Washington, D.C.: U.S. Government Printing Office, 1975). Also, *Federal Register*, Part 3: August 8, 1975, pp. 33526–552.
*Now the Department of Health and Human Services.

quate provision for the monitoring of the consent process, and (d) the pregnant woman has given her informed consent. (Adopted unanimously.)

3. *Nontherapeutic research directed toward the pregnant woman* may be conducted or supported by the Secretary, DHEW, provided such research (a) has been evaluated for possible impact on the fetus, (b) will impose minimal or no risk to the well-being of the fetus, (c) has been approved by existing review procedures with adequate provision for the monitoring of the consent process, (d) special care has been taken to assure that the woman has been fully informed regarding possible impact on the fetus, and (e) the woman has given informed consent. (Adopted unanimously.)

It is further provided that nontherapeutic research directed at the pregnant woman may be conducted or supported (f) only if the father has not objected, both where abortion is not at issue (adopted by a vote of 8 to 1) and where an abortion is anticipated (adopted by a vote of 5 to 4).

4. *Nontherapeutic research directed toward the fetus in utero* [other than research in anticipation of, or during, abortion] may be conducted or supported by the Secretary, DHEW, provided (a) the purpose of such research is the development of important biomedical knowledge that cannot be obtained by alternative means, (b) investigation on pertinent animal models and nonpregnant humans has preceded such research, (c) minimal or no risk to the well-being of the fetus will be imposed by the research, (d) the research has been approved by existing review procedures with adequate provision for the monitoring of the consent process, (e) the informed consent of the mother has been obtained, and (f) the father has not objected to the research. (Adopted unanimously.)

5. *Nontherapeutic research directed toward the fetus in anticipation of abortion* may be conducted or supported by

the Secretary, DHEW, provided such research is carried out within the guidelines for all other nontherapeutic research directed toward the fetus in utero. Such research presenting special problems related to the interpretation or application of these guidelines may be conducted or supported by the Secretary, DHEW, provided such research has been approved by a national ethical review body. (Adopted by a vote of 8 to 1.)

6. *Nontherapeutic research directed toward the fetus during the abortion procedure and nontherapeutic research directed toward the nonviable fetus ex utero* may be conducted or supported by the Secretary, DHEW, provided (a) the purpose of such research is the development of important biochemical knowledge that cannot be obtained by alternative means, (b) investigation on pertinent animal models and nonpregnant humans (when appropriate) has preceded such research, (c) the research has been approved by existing review procedures with adequate provision for the monitoring of the consent process, (d) the informed consent of the mother has been obtained, and (e) the father has not objected to the research; and provided further that (f) the fetus is less than twenty weeks gestational age, (g) no significant procedural changes are introduced into the abortion procedure in the interest of research alone, and (h) no intrusion into the fetus is made which alters the duration of life. Such research presenting special problems related to the interpretation or application of these guidelines may be conducted or supported by the Secretary, DHEW, provided such research has been approved by a national ethical review body. (Adopted by a vote of 8 to 1.)

7. *Nontherapeutic research directed toward the possibly viable infant* may be conducted or supported by the Secretary, DHEW, provided (a) the purpose of such research is the development of important biomedical knowledge that cannot be obtained by alternative means, (b) investigation on per-

tinent animal models and nonpregnant humans (when appropriate) has preceded such research, (c) no additional risk to the well-being of the infant will be imposed by the research, (d) the research has been approved by existing review procedures with adequate provision for the monitoring of the consent process, and (e) informed consent of either parent has been given and neither parent has objected. (Adopted unanimously.)

8. *Review procedures.* Until the Commission makes its recommendations regarding review and consent procedures, the review procedures mentioned above are to be those presently required by the Department of Health, Education, and Welfare. In addition, provision for monitoring the consent process will be required in order to ensure adequacy of the consent process and to prevent unfair discrimination in the selection of research subjects, for all categories of research mentioned above. A national ethical review, as required in Recommendations (5) and (6), shall be carried out by an appropriate body designated by the Secretary, DHEW, until the establishment of the National Advisory Council for the Protection of Subjects of Biomedical and Behavioral Research. In order to facilitate public understanding and the presentation of public attitudes toward special problems reviewed by the national review body, appropriate provision should be made for public attendance and public participation in the national review process. (Adopted unanimously, one abstention.)

9. *Research on the Dead Fetus and Fetal Tissue.* The Commission recommends the use of the dead fetus, fetal tissue and fetal material for research purposes be permitted, consistent with the local law, the Uniform Anatomical Gift Act and commonly held convictions about respect for the dead. (Adopted unanimously, one abstention.)

10. The design and conduct of a nontherapeutic research protocol should not determine recommendations by a physi-

cian regarding the advisability, timing, or method of abortion. (Adopted by a vote of 6 to 2.)

11. Decisions made by a personal physician concerning the health care of a pregnant woman or fetus should not be compromised for research purposes, and when a physician of record is involved in a prospective research protocol, independent medical judgment on these issues is required. In such cases, review panels should assure that procedures for such independent medical judgment are adequate, and all conflict of interest or appearance thereof between appropriate health care and research objectives should be avoided. (Adopted unanimously.)

12. The Commission recommends that research on abortion techniques continue as permitted by law and government regulation. (Adopted by a vote of 6 to 2.)

13. The Commission recommends that attention be drawn to Section 214(d) of the National Research Act (P.L. 93-348), which provides that:

> No individual shall be required to perform or assist in the performance of any part of a health service program or research activity funded in whole or in part by the Secretary of Health, Education, and Welfare if his performance or assistance in the performance of such part of such program or activity would be contrary to his religious beliefs or moral convictions.

(Adopted unanimously.)

14. No inducements, monetary or otherwise, should be offered to procure an abortion for research purposes. (Adopted unanimously.)

15. Research which is supported by the Secretary, DHEW, to be conducted outside the United States should

at the minimum comply in full with the standards and procedures recommended herein. (Adopted unanimously.)

16. The moratorium which is currently in effect should be lifted immediately, allowing research to proceed under current regulations but with the application of the Commission's Recommendations to the review process. All the foregoing Recommendations of the Commission should be implemented as soon as the Secretary, DHEW, is able to promulgate regulations based upon these Recommendations and the public response to them. (Adopted by a vote of 9 to 1.)

Appendix E

The Belmont Report of the National Commission for the Protection of Human Subjects of Biomedical and Behavioral Research

Ethical Principles and Guidelines for Research Involving Human Subjects

Scientific research has produced substantial social benefits. It has also posed some troubling ethical questions. Public attention was drawn to these questions by reported abuses of human subjects in biomedical experiments, especially during the Second World War. During the Nuremberg War Criminal Trials, the Nuremberg Code was drafted as a set of standards for judging physicians and scientists who had conducted biomedical experiments on concentration camp prisoners. This code became the prototype of many later codes[1] intended to assure that research involving human subjects would be carried out in an ethical manner.

The codes consist of rules, some general, others specific,

Federal Regulation Doc. 79-12065, April 18, 1979.

that guide the investigator or the reviewers of research in their work. Such rules often are inadequate to cover complex situations; at times they come in conflict, and they are frequently difficult to interpret or apply. Broader ethical principles will provide a basis on which specific rules may be formulated, criticized and interpreted.

Three principles, or general prescriptive judgments, that are relevant to research involving human subjects are identified in this statement. Other principles may also be relevant. These three are comprehensive, however, and are stated at a level of generalization that should assist scientists, subjects, reviewers, and interested citizens to understand the ethical issues inherent in research involving human subjects. These principles cannot always be applied so as to resolve beyond dispute particular ethical problems. The objective is to provide an analytical framework that will guide the resolution of ethical problems arising from research involving human subjects.

This statement consists of a distinction between research and practice, a discussion of the three basic ethical principles, and remarks about the application of these principles.

BOUNDARIES BETWEEN PRACTICE AND RESEARCH

It is important to distinguish between biomedical and behavioral research, on the one hand, and the practice of accepted therapy on the other, in order to know what activities ought to undergo review for the protection of human subjects of research. The distinction between research and practice is blurred partly because both often occur together (as in research designed to evaluate a therapy) and partly because notable departures from standard practice are often called "experimental" when the terms "experimental" and "research" are not carefully defined.

For the most part, the term "practice" refers to interventions that are designed solely to enhance the well-being of an individual patient or client and that have a reasonable expectation of success. The purpose of medical or behavioral practice is to provide diagnosis, preventive treatment or therapy to particular individuals.[2] By contrast, the term "research" designates an activity designed to test an hypothesis, permit conclusions to be drawn, and thereby to develop or contribute to generalizable knowledge (expressed, for example, in theories, principles, and statements of relationships). Research is usually described in a formal protocol that sets forth an objective and a set of procedures designed to reach that objective.

When a clinician departs in a significant way from standard or accepted practice, the innovation does not, in and of itself, constitute research. The fact that a procedure is "experimental," in the sense of new, untested or different, does not automatically place it in the category of research. Radically new procedures of this description should, however, be made the object of formal research at an early stage in order to determine whether they are safe and effective. Thus, it is the responsibility of medical practice committees, for example, to insist that a major innovation be incorporated into a formal research project.[3]

Research and practice may be carried on together when research is designed to evaluate the safety and efficacy of a therapy. This need not cause any confusion regarding whether or not the activity requires review; the general rule is that if there is any element of research in an activity, that activity should undergo review for the protection of human subjects.

BASIC ETHICAL PRINCIPLES

The expression "basic ethical principles" refers to those general judgments that serve as a basic justification for the many particular ethical prescriptions and evaluations of human actions. Three basic principles, among those generally accepted in our cultural tradition, are particularly relevant to the ethics of research involving human subjects: the principles of respect for persons, beneficence, and justice.

1. **Respect for Persons:** Respect for persons incorporates at least two ethical convictions: first, that individuals should be treated as autonomous agents, and second, that persons with diminished autonomy are entitled to protection. The principle of respect for persons thus divides into two separate moral requirements: the requirement to acknowledge autonomy and the requirement to protect those with diminished autonomy.

An autonomous person is an individual capable of deliberation about personal goals and of acting under the direction of such deliberation. To respect autonomy is to give weight to autonomous persons' considered opinions and choices while refraining from obstructing their actions unless they are clearly detrimental to others. To show lack of respect for an autonomous agent is to repudiate that person's considered judgments, to deny an individual the freedom to act on those considered judgments, or to withhold information necessary to make a considered judgment, when there are no compelling reasons to do so.

However, not every human being is capable of self-determination. The capacity for self-determination matures during an individual's life, and some individuals lose this capacity wholly or in part because of illness, mental disability, or circumstances that severely restrict liberty. Respect for the immature and the incapacitated may require protecting them as they mature or while they are incapacitated.

Some persons are in need of extensive protection, even to the point of excluding them from activities which may harm them; other persons require little protection beyond making sure they undertake activities freely and with awareness of possible adverse consequences. The extent of protection afforded should depend upon the risk of harm and the likelihood of benefit. The judgment that any individual lacks autonomy should be periodically reevaluated and will vary in different situations.

In most cases of research involving human subjects, respect for persons demands that subjects enter into the research voluntarily and with adequate information. In some situations, however, application of the principle is not obvious. The involvement of prisoners as subjects of research provides an instructive example. On the one hand, it would seem that the principle of respect for persons requires that prisoners not be deprived of the opportunity to volunteer for research. On the other hand, under prison conditions they may be subtly coerced or unduly influenced to engage in research activities for which they would not otherwise volunteer. Respect for persons would then dictate that prisoners be protected. Whether to allow prisoners to "volunteer" or to "protect" them presents a dilemma. Respecting persons, in most hard cases, is often a matter of balancing competing claims urged by the principle of respect itself.

2. **Beneficence:** Persons are treated in an ethical manner not only by respecting their decision and protecting them from harm, but also by making efforts to secure their well-being. Such treatment falls under the principle of beneficence. The term "beneficence" is often understood to cover acts of kindness or charity that go beyond strict obligations. In this document, beneficence is understood in a stronger sense, as an obligation. Two general rules have been formulated as complementary expressions of beneficent actions in this sense: (1) do not harm and (2) maximize possible benefits and minimize possible harms.

The Hippocratic maxim "do no harm" has long been a fundamental principle of medical ethics. Claude Bernard extended it to the realm of research, saying that one should not injure one person regardless of the benefits that might come to others. However, even avoiding harm requires learning what is harmful; and, in the process of obtaining this information, persons may be exposed to risk of harm. Further, the Hippocratic Oath requires physicians to benefit their patients "according to their best judgment." Learning what will in fact benefit may require exposing persons to risk. The problem posed by these imperatives is to decide when it is justifiable to seek certain benefits despite the risks involved, and when the benefits should be foregone because of the risks.

The obligations of beneficence affect both individual investigators and society at large, because they extend both to particular research projects and to the entire enterprise of research. In the case of particular projects, investigators and members of their institution are obliged to give forethought to the maximization of benefits and the reduction of risk that might occur from the research investigation. In the case of scientific research in general, members of the larger society are obliged to recognize the longer-term benefits and risks that may result from the improvement of knowledge and from the development of novel medical, psychotherapeutic, and social procedures.

The principle of beneficence often occupies a well-defined justifying role in many areas of research involving human subjects. An example is found in research involving children. Effective ways of treating childhood diseases and fostering health development are benefits that serve to justify research involving children—even when individual research subjects are not direct beneficiaries. Research also makes it possible to avoid the harm that may result from the application of previously accepted routine practices that on closer investigation turn out to be dangerous. But the role of the principle of beneficence is not always so unambiguous. A difficult ethical problem remains, for example, about research that presents more than minimal risk without immediate prospect of direct benefit to the children involved. Some have argued that such research is inadmissible, while others have pointed out that this limit would rule out much research promising great benefit to children in the future. Here again, as with all hard cases, the different claims covered by the principle of beneficence may come into conflict and force difficult choices.

3. **Justice:** Who ought to receive the benefits of research and bear its burdens? This is a question of justice, in the sense of "fairness in distribution" or "what is deserved." An injustice occurs when some benefit to which a person is entitled is denied without good reason or when some burden is imposed unduly. Another way of conceiving the principle of justice is that equals ought to be treated equally. However, this statement requires explication. Who is equal and who is unequal? What considerations justify departure from equal distribution? Almost all commentators allow that distinctions based on experience, age, deprivation, competence, merit, and position do sometimes constitute criteria justifying differential treatment for certain purposes. It is necessary, then, to explain in what respects people should be treated equally. There are several widely accepted formulations of just ways to distribute burdens and benefits. Each formulation mentions some relevant property on the basis of which burdens and benefits should be distributed. These formulations are (1) to each person an equal share, (2) to each person according to individual need, (3) to each person according to individual effort, (4) to each person according to societal contribution, and (5) to each person according to merit.

Questions of justice have long been associated with social practices such as punishment, taxation, and political representation. Until recently these questions have not generally been associated with scientific research. However, they are foreshadowed even in the earliest reflections on the ethics of research involving human subjects. For example, during the nineteenth and early twentieth centuries the burdens of serving as research subjects fell largely upon poor ward patients, while the benefits of improved medical care flowed primarily to private patients. Subsequently, the exploitation of unwilling prisoners as research subjects in Nazi concentration camps was condemned as a particularly flagrant injustice. In this country, in the 1940s, the Tuskegee syphilis study used disadvantaged, rural black men to study the untreated course of a disease that is by no means confined to that population. These subjects were deprived of demonstrably effective treatment in order not to interrupt the project, long after such treatment became generally available.

Against this historical background, it can be seen how conceptions of justice are relevant to research involving human subjects. For example, the selection of research subjects needs to be scrutinized in order to determine whether some classes (e.g., welfare patients, particular racial and ethnic minorities, or persons confined to institutions) are being systematically selected simply because of their easy availability, their compromised position, or their manipulability, rather than for reasons directly related to the problem being studied. Finally, whenever research supported by public funds leads to the development of therapeutic devices and procedures, justice demands both that these not provide advantages only to those who can afford them and that such research should not unduly involve persons from groups unlikely to be among the beneficiaries of subsequent applications of the research.

APPLICATIONS

Applications of the general principles to the conduct of research leads to consideration of the following requirements: informed consent, risk/benefit assessment, and the selection of subjects of research.

1. **Informed Consent:** Respect for persons requires that subjects, to the degree that they are capable, be given the opportunity to choose what shall or shall not happen to them. This opportunity is provided when adequate standards of informed consent are satisfied.

While the importance of informed consent is unquestioned, controversy prevails over the nature and possibility of an informed consent. Nonetheless, there is widespread agreement that the consent process can be analyzed as containing three elements: information, comprehension, and voluntariness.

Information: Most codes of research establish specific items for disclosure intended to assure that subjects are given sufficient information. These items generally include: the research procedure, their purposes, risks and anticipated benefits, alternative procedures (where therapy is involved), and a statement offering the subject the opportunity to ask questions and to withdraw at any time from the research. Additional items have been proposed, including how subjects are selected, the person responsible for the research, etc.

However, a simple listing of items does not answer the question of what the standard should be for judging how much and what sort of information should be provided. One standard frequently invoked in medical practice, namely, the information commonly provided by practitioners in the field or in the locale, is inadequate since research takes place precisely when a common understanding does not exist. Another standard, commonly popular in malpractice law, requires the practitioner to reveal the information that reasonable persons would wish to know in order to make a decision regarding their care. This, too, seems insufficient since the research subject, being in essence a volunteer, may wish to know considerably more about risks gratuitously undertaken than do patients who deliver themselves into the hands of a clinician for needed care. It may be that a standard of "the reasonable volunteer" should be proposed: the extent and nature of in-

formation should be such that persons, knowing that a procedure is neither necessary for their care nor perhaps fully
understood, can decide whether they wish to participate in
the furthering of knowledge. Even when some direct benefit
to them is anticipated, the subjects should understand clearly
the range of risk and the voluntary nature of participation.

A special problem of consent arises where informing subjects of some pertinent aspect of the research is likely to impair
the validity of the research. In many cases, it is sufficient
to indicate to subjects that they are being invited to participate
in research of which some features will not be revealed until
the research is concluded. In all cases of research involving
incomplete disclosure, such research is justified only if it is
clear that (1) incomplete disclosure is truly necessary to accomplish the goals of the research, (2) there are no undis-
closed risks to subjects that are more than minimal, and
(3) there is an adequate plan for debriefing subjects, when
appropriate, and for dissemination of research results to them.
Information about risks should never be withheld for the
purpose of eliciting the cooperation of subjects, and truthful
answers should always be given to direct questions about
the research. Care should be taken to distinguish cases in
which disclosure would destroy or invalidate the research
from cases in which disclosure would simply inconvenience
the investigator.

Comprehension: The manner and context in which information is conveyed is as important as the information itself.
For example, presenting information in a disorganized and
rapid fashion, allowing too little time for consideration or
curtailing opportunities for questioning, all may adversely
affect a subject's ability to make an informed choice.

Because the subject's ability to understand is a function
of intelligence, rationality, maturity, and language, it is necessary to adapt the presentation of the information to the
subject's capacities. Investigators are responsible for ascertaining that the subject has comprehended the information.

While there is always an obligation to ascertain that the information about risks to subjects is complete and adequately comprehended, when the risks are more serious, that obligation increases. On occasion, it may be suitable to give some oral or written tests of comprehension.

Special provisions may need to be made when comprehension is severely limited—for example, by conditions of immaturity or mental disability. Each class of subjects that one might consider as incompetent (e.g., infants and young children, mentally disabled patients, the terminally ill and the comatose) should be considered on its own terms. Even for these persons, however, respect requires giving them the opportunity to choose to the extent they are able, whether or not to participate in research. The objections of these subjects to involvement should be honored, unless the research entails providing them a therapy unavailable elsewhere. Respect for persons also requires seeking the permission of other parties in order to protect the subjects from harm. Such persons are thus respected both by acknowledging their own wishes and by the use of third parties to protect them from harm.

The third parties chosen should be those who are most likely to understand the incompetent subject's situation and to act in that person's best interest. The person authorized to act on behalf of the subject should be given an opportunity to observe the research as it proceeds in order to be able to withdraw the subject from the research, if such action appears in the subject's best interest.

Voluntariness: An agreement to participate in research constitutes a valid consent only if voluntarily given. This element of informed consent requires conditions free of coercion and undue influence. Coercion occurs when an overt threat of harm is intentionally presented by one person to another in order to obtain compliance. Undue influence, by contrast, occurs through an offer of an excessive, unwarranted, inappropriate, or improper reward or other overture in order to obtain compliance. Also, inducements that would ordinarily be acceptable may become undue influences if the subject is especially vulnerable.

Unjustifiable pressures usually occur when persons in positions of authority or commanding influence—especially where possible sanctions are involved—urge a course of action for a subject. A continuum of such influencing factors exists, however, and it is impossible to state precisely where justifiable persuasion ends and undue influence begins. But undue influence would include actions such as manipulating a person's choice through the controlling influence of a close relative and threatening to withdraw health services to which an individual would otherwise be entitled.

2. **Assessment of Risks and Benefits:** The assessment of risks and benefits requires a careful array of relevant data, including, in some cases, alternative ways of obtaining the benefits sought in the research. Thus, the assessment presents both an opportunity and a responsibility to gather systematic and comprehensive information about proposed research. For the investigator, it is a means to examine whether the proposed research is properly designed. For a review committee, it is a method for determining whether the risks that will be presented to subjects are justified. For prospective subjects, the assessment will assist the determination whether or not to participate.

The Nature and Scope of Risks and Benefits: The requirement that research be justified on the basis of a favorable risk/benefit assessment bears a close relation to the principle of beneficence, just as the moral requirement that informed consent be obtained is derived primarily from the principle of respect for persons. The term "risk" refers to a possibility that harm may occur. However, when expressions such as "small risk" or "high risk" are used, they usually refer (often ambiguously), both to the chance (probability) of experiencing a harm and the severity (magnitude) of the envisioned harm.

The term "benefit" is used in the research context to refer

to something of positive value related to health or welfare. Unlike "risk," "benefit" is not a term that expresses probabilities. Risk is properly contrasted with harms rather than risks of harm. Accordingly, so-called risk/benefit assessments are concerned with the probabilities and magnitudes of possible harms and anticipated benefits. Many kinds of possible harms and benefits need to be taken into account. There are, for example, risks of psychological harm, physical harm, legal harm, social harm, and economic harm and the corresponding benefits. While the most likely types of harms to research subjects are those of psychological or physical pain or injury, other possible kinds should not be overlooked.

Risks and benefits of research may affect the individual subjects, the families of the individual subjects, and society at large (or special groups of subjects in society). Previous codes and federal regulations have required that risks to subjects be outweighed by the sum of both the anticipated benefit to the subject, if any, and the anticipated benefit to society of the form of knowledge to be gained from the research. In balancing these different elements, the risks and benefits affecting the immediate research subject will normally carry special weight. On the other hand, interests other than those of the subject may on some occasions be sufficient by themselves to justify the risks involved in the research, so long as the subjects' rights have been protected. Beneficence thus requires that we protect against risk of harm to subjects and also that we be concerned about the loss of the substantial benefits that might be gained from research.

The Systematic Assessment of Risks and Benefits: It is commonly said that benefits and risks must be "balanced" and shown to be "in the favorable ratio." The metaphorical character of these terms draws attention to the difficulty of making precise judgments. Only on rare occasions will quantitative techniques be available for the scrutiny of research protocols. However, the idea of systematic, nonarbitrary analysis of risks and benefits should be emulated insofar as possible. This ideal requires those making decisions about the justifiability of research to be thorough in the accumulation and assessment of information about all aspects of the research, and to consider alternatives systematically. This procedure renders the assessment of research more rigorous and precise, while making communication between review board members and investigators less subject to misinterpretation, misinformation, and conflicting judgments. Thus, there should first be a determination of the validity of the presuppositions of the research; then the nature, probability and magnitude of risk should be distinguished with as much clarity as possible. The method of ascertaining risks should be explicit, especially where there is no alternative to the use of such vague categories as small or slight risk. It should also be determined whether an investigator's estimates of the probability of harm or benefits are reasonable, as judged by known facts or other available studies.

Finally, assessment of the justifiability of research should reflect at least the following considerations: (i) Brutal or inhumane treatment of human subjects is never morally justified. Risks should be reduced to those necessary to achieve the research objective. It should be determined whether it is in fact necessary to use human subjects at all. Risks can perhaps never be entirely eliminated, but it can often be reduced by careful attention to alternative procedures. (iii) When research involves significant risk of serious impairment, review committees should be extraordinarily insistent on the justification of the risk (looking usually to the likelihood of benefit to the subject—or, in some rare cases, to the manifest voluntariness of the participation). (iv) When vulnerable populations are involved in research, the appropriateness of involving them should itself be demonstrated. A number of variables go into such judgments, including the nature and degree of risk, the condition of the particular population involved, and the nature and level of the anticipated benefits. (v) Relevant risks and benefits must be thoroughly arrayed in documents and procedures used in the informed consent process.

3. **Selection of Subjects:** Just as the principle of respect for persons finds expression in the requirements for consent, and the principle of beneficence in risk/benefit assessments, the principle of justice gives rise to moral requirements that there be fair procedures and outcomes in the selection of research subjects.

Justice is relevant to the selection of subjects of research at two levels: the social and the individual. Individual justice in the selection of subjects would require that researchers exhibit fairness: thus, they should not offer potentially beneficial research to some patients who are in their favor or select only "undesirable" persons for risk research. Social justice requires that distinctions be drawn between classes of subjects that ought, and ought not, to participate in any particular kind of research, based on the ability of members of that class to bear burdens and on the appropriateness of placing further burdens on the already burdened persons. Thus, it can be considered a matter of social justice that there is an order of preference in the selection of classes of subjects (e.g., adults before children) and that some classes of potential subjects (e.g., the institutionalized mentally infirm or prisoners) may be involved as research subjects, if at all, only on certain conditions.

Injustice may appear in the selection of subjects, even if individual subjects are selected fairly by investigators and treated fairly in the course of research. Thus injustice arises from social, racial, sexual, and cultural biases institutionalized in society. Thus, even if individual researchers are treating their research subjects fairly, and even if IRBs are taking care to assure that subjects are selected fairly within a particular institution, unjust social patterns may nevertheless appear in the overall distribution of the burdens and benefits of research. Although individual institutions or investigators may not be able to resolve a problem that is pervasive in their social setting, they can consider distributive justice in selecting research subjects.

Some populations, especially institutionalized ones, are already burdened in many ways by their infirmities and environments. When research is proposed that involves risks and does not include a therapeutic component, other, less burdened classes of persons should be called upon first to accept these risks of research, except where the research is directly related to the specific conditions of the class involved. Also, even though public funds for research may often flow in the same direction as public funds for health care, it seems unfair that populations dependent on public health care constitute a pool of preferred research subjects if more advantaged populations are likely to be the recipients of the benefits.

One special instance of injustice results from the involvement of vulnerable subjects. Certain groups, such as racial minorities, the economically disadvantaged, the very sick, and the institutionalized may continually be sought as research subjects, owing to their ready availability in settings where research is conducted. Given their dependent status and their frequently compromised capacity for free consent, they should be protected against the danger of being involved in research solely for administrative convenience, or because they are easy to manipulate as a result of their illness or socioeconomic condition.

NOTES

1. Since 1945, various codes for the proper and responsible conduct of human experimentation in medical research have been adopted by different organizations. The best known of these codes are the Nuremberg Code of 1947, the Helsinki Declaration of 1964 (revised in 1975), and the 1971 guidelines (codified into federal regulation in 1974) issued by the U.S. Department of Health, Education and Welfare. Codes for the conduct of social and behavioral

research have also been adopted, the best known being that of the American Psychological Association, published in 1973.

2. Although practice usually involves intervention designed solely to enhance the well-being of a particular individual, interventions are sometimes applied to one individual for the enhancement of the well-being of another (e.g., blood donations, skin grafts, organ transplants) or an intervention may have the dual purpose of enhancing the well-being of a particular individual, and, at the same time, providing some benefit to others (e.g., vaccination, which protects both the person who is vaccinated and society generally). The fact that some forms of practice have elements other than immediate benefit to the individual receiving an intervention, however, should not confuse the general distinction between research and practice. Even when a procedure applied in practice may benefit some other persons, it remains an intervention designed to enhance the well-being of a particular individual or group of individuals, thus, it is practice and need not be reviewed as research.

3. Because the problems related to social experimentation may differ substantially from those of biomedical and behavioral research, the Commission specifically declines to make any policy determination regarding such research at this time. Rather, the Commission believes that the problem ought to be addressed by one of its successor bodies.

Appendix F

The Foundation of Human Rights

It is within the reciprocal relationship between the individual and society that important issues arise such as human rights and property rights. Since personal behavior impacts upon society and since property is acquired through the social process of the community, one may reasonably argue that the community has some claim as to how behavior is to be managed and how property may be obtained and even how it may be used. Jeremy Waldron has written an in-depth study of the property issue (*Right to Private Property,* Oxford: Clarendon Press, 1988), and C. B. Macpherson has written on the major thinkers crucial to the development of our understanding of property rights (*Property: Mainstream and Critical Positions,* Toronto: University of Toronto Press, 1978).

A vast amount of literature exists concerning these matters, but what is pertinent in regard to my thesis is where the four ethical factors lead us in respect to these topics, irrespective of what I or others may or may not opine. Therefore the following discussion is derived from the fundamental concept of harm-avoidance and outlines the path I believe one should follow in order to resolve the above issues from the ethical point of view.

If we accept the hierarchy of importance of the four factors, then ethically the freedom of the individual to act, to speak, to believe, to move, to emigrate, to isolate self, in essence to do anything he or she may desire, is inviolate as long as harm is not produced. Therefore the right to privacy, the right to his or her talent or property, to be free of restraints, to be free to choose are all inviolate unless significant harm is produced to other individuals, or to society. The determination of what is significant may be difficult, but the attitude which respects the hierarchy of the four factors should help in this determination. These rights must be balanced against the obligations and duties that a person has in respect to society.

Since the approach I have used derives moral factors and subsequently rights and duties from biological reality, it is apparent that the underpinning of rights should theoretically apply to all people regardless of cultural constraints. This is said with full realization of the strength of cultural norms that may be antithetical to the human rights and duties I believe to be valid claims.